T0144659

# BASIC HEALTH PUBLICATIONS USER'S GUIDE

## TO CHRONIC FATIGUE & FIBROMYALGIA

*Learn How to Use Foods and Supplements to Increase Energy Levels and Reduce Pain.*

LAUREL VUKOVIC, M.S.W.

JACK CHALLEM Series Editor

Series Editor: Jack Challem
Editor: Chris Mariadason
Typesetter: Gary A. Rosenberg
Series Cover Designer: Mike Stromberg

Basic Health Publications User's Guides are published by Basic Health Publications, Inc.

# CONTENTS

# THE EPIDEMIC
# OF FATIGUE

It's not an exaggeration to label fatigue as a modern-day epidemic. In fact, fatigue is one of the most common health complaints, and one of the primary reasons for visits to the doctor.

Fatigue can wear many guises, ranging from everyday, run-of-the mill tiredness to incapacitating fatigue that makes it difficult to get out of bed. But no matter how tired you are, or how severe your symptoms may be, you'll find help in this book. You'll learn about fatigue and its causes, as well as the more severe illnesses of chronic fatigue syndrome and fibromyalgia. Chapter 6 outlines the best diet for restoring and maintaining vitality, including specific foods and nutrients that are essential for energy production. In Chapter 7, you'll learn about special nutritional supplements that can dramatically improve your energy and well-being. In Chapters 8 and 9, you'll learn the secrets of tonic herbs that can help to restore your vitality, as well as herbs that help to relieve the symptoms of chronic fatigue and fibromyalgia. In this book, you'll also discover many valuable tips for creating a life of balance that will support you in your quest for improved health and energy.

You've taken an important first step by buying this book. Remember the words of the ancient Chinese philosopher, Lao-tzu, who wisely said, "The journey of a thousand miles begins with a single step." Although you may feel as though you have a long way to go, it's important to be patient with yourself as you embark on your healing journey. You might find it helpful to keep a journal, where you can record your diet, exercise, sleep patterns, and how you are feeling. Keeping track can provide you with valuable information as to what is working, and what isn't. Most of all, remember that your body has a remarkable capacity for healing and rejuvenation.

## CHAPTER 1

# UNDERSTANDING FATIGUE

**A**t the most basic level, fatigue is a powerful feedback tool. If you're feeling tired, your body is telling you that you need to slow down and evaluate how you are living. This includes the obvious factors of diet, exercise, and sleep, as well as the not so obvious factors such as how you manage life stressors.

## Are You Fatigued?

Everyone feels tired at times. It's normal to feel tired after a hard day's work, whether it's mental or physical labor. And it's also normal to feel tired after vigorous exercise. If a good night's sleep or a day of rest and relaxation restores your energy, then you're in good shape and your body is functioning as it should.

Fatigue can be defined as a much deeper, longer-lasting tiredness. If you're fatigued, you feel tired—even exhausted—most of the time. You may feel depressed or irritable, and have difficulties concentrating and accomplishing tasks. It's likely that you lack the energy to do much more than just get through the day, and your enthusiasm has probably waned for activities that you formerly enjoyed.

While fatigue is a symptom of a wide variety of medical conditions, in most cases it's related to lifestyle factors that are within your control. It's important, however, to schedule an evaluation with your healthcare practitioner to rule out underlying physical causes such as anemia, low thyroid function, and diabetes.

## The Primary Causes of Fatigue

Because there are many underlying causes of fatigue, it's helpful to identify which, if any, are contributing to your exhaustion.

Some of the primary reasons for fatigue include dietary factors (nutritional deficiencies, food allergies, and dietary stressors such as caffeine), sleep disorders, lack of exercise (or too much exercise), overworking, emotional stress, low thyroid function, hypoglycemia, and adrenal weakness. All of these factors are explored in depth in this book.

One thing is certain: the world today moves at a faster pace than ever, and most of us feel compelled to try to keep up. Although the natural rhythm of life calls for times of activity balanced with times of rest, few people schedule sufficient time for rest. For example, although most people function best on about eight hours of sleep per night, it's the rare person who meets their sleep needs on a regular basis. Sleeping in on weekends to try to remedy a sleep deficit only makes the problem worse, because doing so further disrupts the body's metabolic clock. Whether you're staying up late working or partying or simply seduced by late-night television, missing out on sleep is one of the most common, and overlooked, causes of fatigue.

In addition, few people take the time to eat relaxed, nutritious meals. Instead, the norm is to grab a quick meal from the nearest fast food drive-thru, or to collapse in front of the television with a microwave dinner. If you're subsisting on a diet of processed foods, your body isn't getting the nutrients it needs to create fuel for your cells. Taking the time for a relaxed meal provides a respite during the day to slow down and nourish not only your body, but your spirit.

## How to Get Started

Once you've seen your doctor and ruled out any underlying conditions that might be causing fatigue, you can get started with the suggestions in this book. Begin with the dietary recommendations in Chapter 6, which will furnish your body with the nutrients it needs to create energy. Make sure to avoid the primary energy zappers: caffeine, sugar, refined carbohydrates, and excessive alcohol. You can rebuild your energy more quickly by providing your body with concentrated nutritional supplements and energy-enhancing tonic herbs. While they can't make up for an unhealthy diet, supplements and tonic herbs play an essential role in building vitality. While you're attending to your diet, also begin following the suggestions in Chapter 10 to ensure that you're getting a good night's sleep. As your energy begins to improve, start a gentle exercise program, which will further increase your vitality. Be careful not to overextend yourself, though, to avoid creating fatigue. And finally, to help stress-proof your life and enhance your overall well-being, follow the suggestions for stress management and relaxation in Chapters 5 and 10.

## CHAPTER 2

# CHRONIC FATIGUE SYNDROME

The tiredness associated with chronic fatigue syndrome, also known as chronic fatigue immune dysfunction syndrome (CFIDS), is different from the ordinary, garden-variety fatigue that everyone experiences after a long day at work or a session of unaccustomed physical activity. The earliest and most significant indication of this debilitating condition is overwhelming fatigue and a lack of stamina that makes it difficult to engage in normal life activities. The fatigue often appears suddenly, and may be continual or intermittent. In addition, even a good night's sleep doesn't relieve the tiredness.

## The Symptoms of Chronic Fatigue

A wide range of symptoms characterizes this debilitating illness; while some people experience only a handful of symptoms, others are plagued by many. The most prominent symptom, of course, is severe exhaustion, which is not alleviated by sleep or rest. Other telltale symptoms are muscle and joint achiness, persistent sore throat, frequent headaches, and tender lymph nodes. The most common symptoms of CFIDS have been described as being similar to having a bad case of the flu. But instead of the illness running its course in a week or two, the symp-

**CFIDS**
*Chronic fatigue immune dysfunction syndrome; a debilitating, chronic illness characterized by severe exhaustion.*

toms persist for six months or more. In addition, emotional and mental symptoms, such as depression and difficulties with concentration, often accompany CFIDS.

One of the reasons that CFIDS is such a puzzling disorder is that the symptoms and their severity often vary so markedly from one person to the next. Symptoms may occur only intermittently, which can be confusing for both the sufferer and for healthcare practitioners attempting to treat the illness. Because many of the symptoms of CFIDS are not apparent to outside observers, it can be difficult for patients to accurately convey to others the severity of their disorder.

In addition to the most common symptoms, CFIDS can cause cognitive disturbances, such as fuzzy thinking, impairment of judgment, and short-term memory disturbances. Psychological problems frequently accompany CFIDS, and include depression, anxiety, irritability, mood swings, and panic attacks. Symptoms of CFIDS can arise in any system of the body and may include irritable bowel syndrome (diarrhea, constipation, and gas), allergies, hypersensitivity (to sounds, odors, chemicals, or medications), irregular heartbeat, chest pains, shortness of breath, lightheadedness, dizziness, fainting, tingling or burning sensations in the extremities, muscle twitches, chills or night sweats, low-grade fever or low body temperature, ringing in the ears, visual disturbances (sensitivity to light, blurry vision, frequent need for prescription changes), and menstrual problems, including PMS and endometriosis.

With the wide-range of symptoms that can be associated with CFIDS, it's no surprise that the condition is challenging for both patients and health practitioners.

## The Prevalence of Chronic Fatigue Syndrome

When chronic fatigue syndrome was first recognized in the early 1980s, it was somewhat derogatorily dubbed "yuppie flu," because the people seeking help were primarily well-educated, affluent women in their thirties and forties. But in reality, there have been similar illnesses recorded as early as the late 1800s that have affected people of all ages, races, and economic backgrounds. For more than 100 years, doctors have attempted to diagnose and put a name to this mysterious and complicated syndrome.

In the late nineteenth century, Dr. George Beard, an American neurologist, came up with the name neurasthenia for a condition characterized by general fatigue, irritability, lack of concentration, and anxiety. A few of the other attempts at explaining the constellation of symptoms that characterize CFIDS have included hypoglycemia (low blood sugar), multiple chemical sensitivity, candidiasis (an overgrowth of yeast throughout the body), and chronic Epstein-Barr virus.

In the late 1980s, the Centers for Disease Control attempted to come up with a standard way of defining the syndrome now known as CFIDS. A group of experts put together a definition of symptoms that was published in the March 1988 issue of *Annals of Internal Medicine*. They called the illness "chronic fatigue syndrome" (CFS), and provided a framework for the further study and evaluation of patients suffering from this disorder. After several years of use the criteria was reevaluated by a group of international CFS experts; the revision was published in December 1994 in *Annals of Internal Medicine*. Today, CFS is also known as myalgic encephalomyelitis, postviral fatigue syndrome, and perhaps most commonly, as chronic fatigue immune dysfunction syndrome.

Because of the challenges inherent in diagnosing CFIDS, it is grossly underdiagnosed. No specific laboratory test has been developed to conclusively identify CFIDS, but the Centers for Disease Control estimate that approximately 500,000 people in the United States are affected by the disease. Some other estimates run even higher. In a study reported in *Archives of Internal Medicine* in 1999, researchers at DePaul University estimated that CFIDS affects approximately 800,000 people in the United States. In addition, close to 90 percent of patients have not been diagnosed and are therefore not receiving appropriate care.

CFIDS tends to affect women almost three times more frequently than men, which is consistent with the occurrence of other autoimmune diseases such as multiple sclerosis and lupus. And although CFIDS occurs more commonly in adults, children and adolescents are also affected by the illness.

## Diagnosing Chronic Fatigue Syndrome

Many people first notice symptoms of CFIDS following a bout with a severe cold, flu, mononucleosis, bronchitis, or hepatitis. Intense, prolonged stress can also trigger the onset of symptoms. While some people fall prey to CFIDS suddenly, in others the illness takes months to develop, with no clearly defined precipitating factor. For the majority of people, the symptoms of CFIDS peak fairly early in the illness, and then tend to come and go.

One of the reasons that chronic fatigue syndrome is underdiagnosed is that it is a challenging illness for physicians to definitively diagnose.

Because there is no diagnostic test specifically for CFIDS, healthcare providers must rule out a variety of other illnesses that share a similar constellation of symptoms. For example, lupus, Lyme disease, hypothyroidism, and multiple chemical sensitivities share some of the same symptoms. The diagnostic process is often time-consuming, challenging, and expensive.

The definition of CFIDS outlined in 1994 provides a helpful tool for evaluation. The criteria for a diagnosis of CFIDS require that four of eight primary symptoms be present, along with fatigue that has interfered with physical, mental, social, and educational activities; both the fatigue and the symptoms must have been present for at least six months. It's important for both doctors and patients to realize that many people with CFIDS experience more than just the eight symptoms outlined by the case definition. Reaching a diagnosis of CFIDS may take months, or even years. It often takes a significant amount of testing, trials of various medications, and numerous physician appointments to finally arrive at a diagnosis.

## Treatment Protocols for Chronic Fatigue

For most people, an effective treatment program for chronic fatigue involves a comprehensive approach to rebuilding health, alleviating symptoms, and restoring energy and vitality. The process can take months, or even years, and it's important to be patient and persistent in your quest for health. In general, therapy for CFIDS entails dietary and lifestyle modifications, specific nutritional and herbal supplements, and supportive therapies to help relieve symptoms and restore vitality. In the following chapters, you'll find the information you need to create your own healing program.

Engaging the help of a healthcare practitioner who is sympathetic to your condition and knowledgeable in the treatment of chronic fatigue immune dysfunction syndrome can be extremely helpful in your healing process.

## CHAPTER 3

# FIBROMYALGIA

**F**ibromyalgia and chronic fatigue syndrome have a lot in common. They share many of the same characteristics, and both have puzzled doctors and researchers for decades. Because fibromyalgia presents many of the same symptoms as CFIDS, the two conditions can be difficult to separate. Both are characterized by a wide variety of physical and emotional symptoms, but the primary identifying factor in fibromyalgia is widespread muscle pain, with specific tender points on various parts of the body.

## What Is Fibromyalgia?

**Fibromyalgia**
*A chronic illness characterized by fatigue and widespread muscle pain of unknown origin.*

Originally thought to be caused by inflammation of the connective tissues, this complex syndrome was first described in medical literature in 1904, when it was called fibrositis. For many years, it was regarded as the most common type of acute and chronic rheumatism.

But it wasn't until the mid-1980s that researchers began to seriously research the painful and disabling condition and renamed it fibromyalgia (*myo* means muscle; *algia* means pain). Fibromyalgia is a complicated disease. Like chronic fatigue syndrome, fibromyalgia is often misdiagnosed, misunderstood, and in many cases, inappropriately treated.

It's estimated that fibromyalgia afflicts some-where between 2 to 4 percent of Americans and affects primarily women (some researchers be-lieve that this statistic reflects the fact that men don't seek help for pain as readily as do women). Today, fibromyalgia is recognized as the second most common form of arthritis (osteoarthritis being the most common).

## Diagnosing Fibromyalgia

Fibromyalgia, like chronic fatigue syndrome, is dif-ficult to diagnose. While other forms of arthritis can be medically verified—for example, inflam-matory forms of arthritis, such as rheumatoid arthritis, show up in blood tests, and degenera-tive forms of arthritis, such as osteoarthritis, show up on x-rays—there are as yet no laboratory tests that can diagnose fibromyalgia. Because of this, those who suffer from fibromyalgia may confront the same skepticism from conventional medical practitioners as do those suffering from chronic fatigue syndrome.

The current consensus is that although fibro-myalgia defies diagnosis with conventional med-ical tests, the condition is, in fact, real. In 1990, the American College of Rheumatologists gave fibromyalgia an official medical definition: the presence of widespread chronic pain for at least three months, with tenderness in at least eleven of eighteen specific points in all four quadrants of the body (upper right, upper left, lower right, and lower left). The problem with these criteria is that the experience of pain is subjective, and ten-der points tend to be more painful on some days than on others. Therefore, the accurate diagnosis of fibromyalgia depends primarily upon a thor-ough case history and the exclusion of other con-ditions that may be causing symptoms.

## Symptoms of Fibromyalgia

One of the challenges in diagnosing fibromyalgia is that symptoms tend to come and go, and the clusters of symptoms vary from person to person. However, muscle fatigue, pain, stiffness, and tender points are always present. The pain and stiffness is often most pronounced in the morning, but may ease somewhat as the day progresses. Cold temperatures, strenuous exercise, and repetitive movements (such as scrubbing a floor) intensify pain and stiffness, while stretching, massage, and the application of heat (such as soaking in a hot bath) provide relief.

One of the primary characteristics of fibromyalgia is abnormal tenderness at specific sites (called tender points or trigger points) in the muscles of the arms, legs, back, and chest when moderate pressure is applied. These eighteen points (actually nine pairs of points) are located within the muscles, or at the points where ligaments attach muscles to bones. Additional common symptoms of fibromyalgia include fatigue that significantly interferes with the activities of daily life, difficulties sleeping, waking up tired even after sufficient sleep, anxiety or depression, digestive disturbances, chronic headaches, Raynaud's syndrome, tingling sensations in the extremities, temporomandibular joint pain (TMJ), and difficulties concentrating.

While fibromyalgia doesn't cause actual joint damage or deformity (as do osteoarthritis and rheumatoid arthritis), it often seriously hinders normal functioning. Symptoms can last for weeks or months, mysteriously get better for a while, and then reappear.

## The Causes of Fibromyalgia

No one knows for sure what causes fibromyalgia.

Many times, the first symptoms of fibromyalgia appear after a traumatic incident, such as an auto accident or a sports injury. A severe viral infection—such as a nasty flu—is also a common precipitating factor; some researchers think that the onset of fibromyalgia is triggered when a virus causes damage at the cellular level. Long-standing nutritional deficiencies, food allergies, exposure to toxic environmental chemicals, and emotional stressors all are thought to play a role in the development of fibromyalgia by interfering with the body's ability to maintain homeostasis.

**Homeostasis** *The complex biochemical processes through which the body maintains balance.*

Whatever the precipitating factor, many researchers believe that fibromyalgia is ultimately caused by an imbalance in brain chemicals that are linked to mood and sleep. The majority of people who suffer from fibromyalgia experience sleep difficulties, including problems falling asleep, waking during the night or early morning hours, and not feeling rested even after sufficient sleep. It's a vicious cycle, because sleep disturbances exacerbate the symptoms of fibromyalgia, and fibromyalgia disrupts sleep. Sleep— especially a period of deep sleep called delta phase sleep— is the time when the body performs restorative activities, such as the repair of muscle tissue. Studies of people with fibromyalgia have shown that they don't obtain sufficient delta sleep, which results in fatigue, morning grogginess, impaired concentration, and irritability. A lack of restorative sleep also results in a reduced output of hormones by the pituitary gland, especially growth hormone, which stimulates tissue repair, and melatonin, which regulates the body's sleep/wake cycles.

## Treatment for Fibromyalgia

Conventional treatments for fibromyalgia often rely on antidepressants, tranquilizers and sedatives for sleep, anti-inflammatory drugs, and muscle relaxants. Interestingly, low dosages of antidepressants can help to relieve fibromyalgia symptoms, even when the dosages given are too low for relieving depression. This may be because antidepressants help to improve sleep, which provides the body with an opportunity for tissue repair.

Many of the symptoms of fibromyalgia are similar to those of chronic fatigue syndrome, with the primary difference being the muscle pain that is specific to fibromyalgia. As with chronic fatigue, healing from fibromyalgia involves dietary and lifestyle modifications, specific nutritional and herbal supplements, and supportive therapies to help relieve symptoms. In the following chapters, you'll find the information you need to create your own healing program. The process of healing from fibromyalgia can take a long time, and you'll probably experience some ups and downs in your journey. As with chronic fatigue syndrome, it's important to be patient and persistent, and to engage the help of a supportive and knowledgeable healthcare practitioner.

## CHAPTER 4

# HIDDEN CAUSES OF FATIGUE

**U**ncovering the cause of fatigue can be complicated because there's often more than one factor involved. Because many fatigue syndromes are intertwined, it's important to consider all possibilities; it's not uncommon to suffer from hypothyroidism and hypoglycemia as well as chronic fatigue syndrome or fibromyalgia at the same time, for example. The conditions in this chapter are some of the most common conditions to consider in treating fatigue.

## Hypoglycemia

One of the most common causes of fatigue is hypoglycemia, or as it's more commonly known, low blood sugar. Other symptoms of this widespread condition include irritability, headaches, dizziness, shakiness, and mental fogginess. These are accompanied by cravings for sugar or refined carbohydrates.

## What Is Hypoglycemia?

For proper mental and physical functioning, glucose has to be constantly available in the bloodstream. In addition, blood-glucose levels have to be maintained within a fairly narrow range. Because glucose is the fuel that powers the brain and body, when blood sugar falls too low, hypoglycemic symptoms result.

The task of maintaining stable blood sugar levels is accomplished by the combined efforts of the pancreas, liver, and adrenal glands. The pancreas monitors blood sugar levels, the liver stores and releases glucose as needed, and the adrenal glands get involved when quick energy is needed, such as in times of stress. Emotional or physical stressors—including rapid drops in blood sugar levels—trigger the adrenals to release adrenaline, a hormone that speeds up the metabolism of glucose. This provides the body with the immediate energy it needs to cope with the stressor.

The body's blood sugar regulating system works well, unless it is exhausted by a diet high in sugar and refined carbohydrates. Because sugar and refined carbohydrates are quickly absorbed into the bloodstream, blood glucose soars. The pancreas scrambles to normalize blood sugar levels by secreting insulin, which causes blood sugar levels to drop. Obviously, this sets the stage for a vicious cycle: Hypoglycemic symptoms create the craving for sugar and refined carbohydrates, which provide a temporary feeling of relief but then quickly result in plummeting blood sugar levels, which again create the need for sugar and refined carbohydrates.

In conventional medical thinking, hypoglycemia is a rare condition that is caused by insulin overdose, which can occur in diabetics, or as the result of a disease such as a pancreatic tumor; this type of hypoglycemia is called "functional hypoglycemia." But the symptoms of hypoglycemia occur in many people who do not suffer from an organic disease. This type of hypoglycemia is referred to as "reactive hypoglycemia," and occurs about two to three hours after a meal, particularly a meal that contains sugar or refined carbohydrates. For most people, modifications in diet and specific

**Hypoglycemia**
*Also called low blood sugar; energy and mood swings caused by eating refined carbohydrates.*

nutritional supplements can help to restore healthy organ function and blood sugar control.

## Dietary Help for Hypoglycemia

Obviously, eliminating sugars and refined carbohydrates is essential for controlling blood sugar levels. It's best to avoid all forms of sugar, including sucrose, glucose, maltose, corn syrup, honey, maple syrup, and molasses. Cookies, candy, and ice cream are obvious sources of concentrated sugars, but many other processed foods, such as salad dressings, pasta sauces, and dry cereals, often contain surprisingly large amounts of added sugars. Because refined carbohydrates—such as breads and pastas made from white flour—have the same effect as simple sugars in the body, they should also be avoided. In addition, caffeine and alcohol both contribute to the problem of hypoglycemia. The stimulating effects of caffeine temporarily increase energy, but tax the adrenal glands. Alcohol impairs the body's ability to use glucose and stimulates the release of insulin, which causes blood sugar levels to plummet.

In lieu of refined sugars, satisfy your cravings for sweets with moderate amounts of fresh fruits and sweet vegetables such as yams, carrots, and winter squash. Choose whole-grain breads, cereals, pastas, and other complex carbohydrates such as brown rice, quinoa, and oatmeal instead of refined products. Many complex carbohydrates are good sources of soluble fiber, which slows the digestion and absorption of carbohydrates and prevents rapid increases in blood sugar. To take advantage of the fiber in carbohydrates, it's important to eat foods in their whole form as much as possible—for example, eat an apple instead of drinking apple juice.

To stabilize blood sugar levels, it's essential to include plenty of high-quality proteins and healthful fats in your diet. Protein is necessary for the proper functioning of the adrenal glands, pancreas, and liver. Because protein doesn't stimulate insulin release, it helps to stabilize blood-sugar levels and curbs cravings for high-carbohydrate foods. Good protein sources include chicken, turkey, fish, and eggs. Healthful fats, such as extra-virgin olive oil, and the fats found in avocados, raw nuts, and olives, also help to maintain stable blood sugar and prevent cravings for simple carbohydrates.

To provide your body with a steady supply of fuel, it's helpful to eat frequent, small meals rather than two or three large meals during the day. Avoid skipping meals or going for more than two or three hours without eating. Try to eat meals at regular times, and plan to eat three meals a day, plus mid-morning, mid-afternoon, and evening snacks. In addition, be sure to get regular exercise. Moderate exercise improves the ability of the cells to respond to insulin and to absorb glucose. The more fit you are, the more responsive your cells will be to insulin, which helps to keep blood sugar under control.

## Supplements and Herbs for Hypoglycemia

One of the most helpful supplements for keeping blood sugar levels stable is the trace mineral chromium. Although it's only needed by the body in tiny amounts, it plays an essential role in how efficiently insulin is used by the cells. Chromium improves the sensitivity of cells to insulin, which helps to keep blood sugar on an even keel and reduces cravings for sugar and refined carbohydrates. Take 200–600 micrograms of chromium in the form of chromium picolinate daily.

Siberian ginseng (*Eleutherococcus senticosus*)

is one of the best herbs for treating hypoglycemia. An excellent overall tonic, Siberian ginseng increases energy by bolstering adrenal function and helps to stabilize blood sugar levels. Take an extract standardized for eleutherosides, approximately 250 milligrams twice daily for three months, with a two-week break before resuming the dosage. Siberian ginseng can be taken indefinitely when used in this way. It generally takes a couple of months to notice the benefits, but you should then be aware of a slow, steady increase in energy. For more information on Siberian ginseng, see Chapter 8.

An herbal tea made from burdock root (*Arctium lappa*), dandelion root (*Taraxacum officinale*), and licorice root (*Glycyrrhiza glabra*) can also help to regulate blood sugar levels. Burdock and dandelion both improve liver function, and licorice strengthens adrenal function and has a naturally sweet flavor that does not increase blood sugar. Because licorice root can potentially increase blood pressure, consult your doctor before using it if you have hypertension. To make a tea that can help to balance blood sugar, simmer one tablespoon each of burdock, dandelion, and licorice in four cups of water in a covered pot for fifteen minutes. Remove from heat and steep an additional fifteen minutes. Strain, and drink up to three cups a day.

## Hypothyroidism

Another common underlying cause of persistent fatigue is hypothyroidism, or low thyroid function. In fact, chronic fatigue and fibromyalgia share many of the same symptoms as hypothyroidism, and the conditions may be connected. Because

**Hypothyroidism**
*Low thyroid function caused by diminished output of thyroid hormone; fatigue is a telltale symptom.*

most conventional doctors rely solely on blood tests, many cases of low thyroid function go undiagnosed, and symptoms are attributed to aging or stress.

## What Is Hypothyroidism?

The thyroid gland, a butterfly-shaped gland that wraps around the windpipe directly below the Adam's apple, is part of the endocrine system. This small gland plays a critical role in controlling metabolism and energy production. When the thyroid isn't functioning up to par, metabolism slows down—sometimes to barely a crawl. Symptoms include fatigue, depression, weight gain, difficulties concentrating, cold hands and feet, constipation, dry skin, hair loss, and muscle and joint pain.

## Diagnosing Hypothyroidism

Treating hypothyroidism is simple, but diagnosing the problem is often challenging. Mild hypothyroidism, which can cause debilitating symptoms, often doesn't show up on standard blood tests. A basal body temperature test is a much more sensitive and accurate measure of thyroid function, and it's something you can easily do at home.

Basal body temperature, the temperature of your body at rest, is a good indication of metabolic rate, which is regulated by the thyroid gland. If the thyroid gland isn't producing enough hormones, metabolism slows down, causing the unpleasant symptoms characteristic of hypothyroidism. To measure your basal body temperature, you'll need to take your temperature as soon as you awaken in the morning, before you get out of bed.

**Basal Body Temperature**
*The temperature of your body at rest; an accurate measure of thyroid function.*

To obtain an accurate reading, it's important to make as little movement as possible. Shake the thermometer down to below 95 degrees Fahrenheit before you go to sleep at night, and when you awaken, place the thermometer in your armpit. Rest and keep your eyes closed for ten minutes, and then record the temperature. (If you have a digital thermometer, the reading will be almost instantaneous and you won't need to lie still for ten minutes.) Repeat this procedure for three consecutive mornings. Because of natural variations in body temperature caused by hormonal fluctuations, menstruating women should perform this test on the second, third, and fourth days of menstruation. Your basal body temperature should be between 97.6 and 98.2 degrees Fahrenheit. A reading lower than this may indicate low thyroid function, especially if you also have other symptoms of hypothyroidism.

## Treatment for Hypothyroidism

In some cases, particularly with very mild cases of hypothyroidism, you might be able to provide enough support to your thyroid gland with a thyroid supplement that contains natural thyroid extract plus nutrients that specifically support thyroid function, such as zinc, iodine, and tyrosine. These combination supplements are commonly available at natural foods stores.

If you have mild hypothyroidism, you might also benefit from herbal treatments, which provide a gentle boost to thyroid function. It's important to work with a qualified herbalist or other health practitioner if you are attempting to treat hypothyroidism with herbs. Guggul (*Commiphora mukul*) is an Ayurvedic herb that has been found to increase levels of thyroid hormones. A typical dosage is 500 mg of guggul, standardized to contain 2.5 percent of guggulsterones (considered to be the active ingredient), three times daily with meals. Ashwagandha (*Withania somnifera*) is an Ayurvedic tonic herb that has been shown in animal studies to also increase levels of thyroid hormones. Ashwagandha is discussed in detail in Chapter 8.

In many cases, hypothyroidism requires supplemental thyroid hormones, which are available only by prescription from a health practitioner. Most doctors assess thyroid function with blood tests, which measure levels of two thyroid hormones, thyroxine (T4) and triiodothyronine (T3), as well as thyroid-stimulating hormone (TSH). TSH is secreted by the pituitary gland, and high levels of this hormone indicate that the thyroid gland isn't working properly. The most popular conventional treatment for hypothyroidism is a synthetic version of thyroid hormone called Synthroid (levothyroxine), which is equivalent to T4. The rationale behind this approach is that T4 is converted to T3 in the body. Many alternative practitioners prefer using desiccated thyroid, a natural preparation made from dried pig thyroid that contains both T3 and T4.

Even if your blood tests come back within normal ranges, you still may be suffering from subclinical hypothyroidism, defined as low thyroid function that doesn't show up on tests. Again, basal temperature may be a more accurate indication of how well your thyroid gland is functioning. Many health practitioners are now realizing that symptoms of low thyroid function—even if tests indicate that the thyroid is functioning normally—present a valid reason to supplement with thyroid hormone.

## Factors That Affect Thyroid Function

A variety of factors influence thyroid function and should be considered when treating hypothyroidism. If you are taking thyroid supplements, you should take them first thing in the morning on an empty stomach, preferably at least one hour before eating. This ensures maximum absorption, and prevents the possibility of other nutrients interfering with the hormone. Because calcium and iron supplements negatively affect thyroid absorption, you shouldn't take calcium or iron within four hours of taking thyroid. This also applies to calcium-fortified foods, such as orange juice with added calcium.

Certain foods have a suppressive effect on thyroid function, and should be avoided if you suffer from hypothyroidism. Millet, soy, peanuts, pine nuts, and cruciferous vegetables such as broccoli, Brussels sprouts, cabbage, cauliflower, kale, radishes, and turnips contain compounds called goitrogens that prevent the thyroid gland from using iodine to make T4. These foods primarily are problematic if they are eaten raw; cooking appears to inactivate the goitrogens. However, if you have been diagnosed with hypothyroidism, you probably shouldn't eat large amounts of these foods.

## CHAPTER 5

# HOW TO
# REDUCE STRESS
# AND GAIN ENERGY

**S**tress, especially chronic, unresolved stress, takes a significant toll on your physical and emotional well-being—in fact, as much as 90 percent of all illness is stress related. Learning healthy ways of coping with stress is essential for overcoming fatigue, chronic fatigue, and fibromyalgia.

## The Body's Response to Stress

Under stress, the autonomic nervous system is aroused, which speeds up heart rate and breathing, raises blood pressure, dumps stored sugars in the form of glucose into the bloodstream, and increases levels of stress hormones such as adrenaline and cortisol, which are produced by the adrenal glands. Dubbed the "fight-or-flight response," this reaction is an automatic, life-saving instinct that provides the energy and strength to deal with dangerous situations.

> **Autonomic Nervous System**
> *The part of the nervous system that controls involuntary functions such as heart rate and breathing.*

Our bodies, however, don't distinguish between life-threatening danger and stressors such as job pressures and financial worries. The resulting flood of stress hormones causes fatigue, depression, anxiety, insomnia, headaches, irritability, muscle tension, and digestive disorders. Conventional medicine relies on tranquilizers for relieving stress, but these drugs have serious side effects, including mental confusion, grogginess, and rebound anxiety. Luckily, in most cases, there's no need to turn to drugs. Lifestyle modifications—including diet, exercise, and rest—strengthen your resistance to stress. And simple relaxation techniques, such as breathing exercises and meditation, provide concrete skills for coping with stressors.

## Dietary Help for Stress

A nutrient-rich diet is essential for building a strong foundation that will help your body cope with stressful situations. Follow the guidelines in Chapter 6 for a health-enhancing diet. If you are feeling stressed, it's especially important to avoid food stressors such as caffeine, alcohol, sugar, and refined carbohydrates.

Caffeine is one of the primary offenders in triggering feelings of stress and anxiety. Even in small amounts, caffeine commonly causes restlessness, heart palpitations, headaches, and insomnia. Eliminate all sources of caffeine, including coffee, black tea, chocolate, cocoa, caffeinated soft drinks, coffee-flavored ice cream and candies, and over-the-counter medications that contain caffeine. It's also best to avoid alcohol if you're under stress. Although it is often used as a relaxant, alcohol can intensify anxiety through its effects on the endocrine and nervous systems.

Sugar and refined carbohydrates are another significant source of dietary stress. Because they are quickly absorbed into the bloodstream, they cause rapid increases in blood sugar levels, followed by equally rapid declines. This roller-coaster effect taxes the adrenal glands, causes fatigue, and is the primary factor in reactive hypoglycemia. (See Chapter 4 for more information on hypoglycemia.) Choose complex carbohydrates instead, which are found abundantly in vegetables, fruits, legumes, and whole grains. These healthful whole-food sugars help to stabilize blood sugar levels and supply steady energy to your body and your brain.

Eating plenty of fresh vegetables and fruits also ensures a rich supply of potassium, which is essential for strengthening the adrenal glands. The ideal dietary ratio for adrenal health is five times the amount of potassium to sodium; however, most people consume only half as much potassium as sodium in their daily diet. Reduce your sodium intake by cutting back on salty snack foods such as chips, and eliminate the added use of salt at the table. In addition, eat at least seven servings of vegetables and fruits daily, which typically contain at least one hundred times more potassium than sodium.

Other nutrients that are important for supporting adrenal health are vitamin C, pantothenic acid (vitamin $B_5$), vitamin $B_6$, magnesium, and zinc. Many fruits and vegetables, including broccoli, cantaloupe, grapefruit, red peppers, and strawberries, are excellent sources of vitamin C. Vitamin $B_5$ is found in avocados, chicken, eggs, mushrooms, salmon, and yogurt. Sources of vitamin $B_6$ include lentils, potatoes, sweet potatoes, tempeh, and tuna. Zinc occurs abundantly in black beans, mussels, oysters, pumpkin seeds, and sesame seeds. Magnesium-rich foods include almonds, corn, halibut, tofu, and peas. In addition to eating foods that supply these important stress-combating nutrients, it's a good idea to take a high-potency vitamin and mineral supplement (along with additional supplements if necessary) to supply 500 mg of vitamin C, 50–100 mg of the B-complex vitamins, 400 mg of magnesium, and 25 mg of zinc.

## Relieve Stress with Exercise

Regular exercise is one of the best and quickest ways to relieve tension and to increase your body's resistance to stress. Exercise metabolizes the stress-producing hormones that are secreted by the adrenal glands and also triggers the release of natural stress-relieving compounds called endorphins. If you suffer from chronic fatigue or fibromyalgia, it's important not to engage in exercise that is overly strenuous. But even gentle movement, such as yoga or tai chi, can help to alleviate stress.

Practicing the technique of mindfulness while you are exercising increases the stress-relieving benefits. Learning to exercise in a mindful way allows you to gain a better perspective on stress, and enables you to more quickly achieve a state of calmness.

A low-intensity, rhythmic aerobic exercise that doesn't require much concentration is best for practicing mindful exercise—walking is perfect. Choose a simple prayer or phrase that you find calming; for example, "All is well" or "I am relaxed." As you walk, recite your chosen word or phrase over and over, in rhythm with your steps. Repeating a word or phrase helps to quiet the mind, and allows you to concentrate on your body's movement and on your breathing. When your mind wanders, gently bring your attention back to your steps and your mindful phrase. The more you practice, the easier mindful exercise becomes, until it becomes natural to leave your worries behind.

## Practice Relaxation to Reduce Stress

Learning to relax is essential for relieving stress. When you take the time to relax, stress hormones subside and your body has the opportunity to calm down. Deep breathing exercises, meditation, and visualization are some of the simple, yet powerful ways that train your body and mind to relax. Relaxation exercises are easy to learn, and can be practiced anywhere. Choose a technique that appeals to you (see Chapter 10 for suggestions) and set aside at least ten minutes every day to practice.

Conscious breathing exercises are especially helpful for relieving stress and anxiety, because deep, relaxed breathing triggers the body to immediately relax. Conscious breathing exercises take only a few minutes a day, and the more you practice them, the easier it will be to use your breath as a tool for relaxation.

## Simplify Your Life

Simplifying your life is a concrete way of reducing stress. Many times, we are driven by time pressures, schedules packed with activities, and lives overflowing with obligations that require an enormous amount of energy to maintain. If you suffer from fatigue, chronic fatigue, or fibromyalgia, simplifying your life will allow you the time, space, and energy you need to heal.

One of the primary stressors for many people in our society is time pressure. It's important to set priorities, and to accept that there is only so much that you can accomplish in one day. This is especially important if you suffer from fatigue or pain. If you frequently feel time pressured, take a thoughtful look at how you are structuring your life. Decide what is really important to you, schedule less than you think you can do, ask other people for help, and practice letting the rest go. In addition, it's essential that you take time for yourself each day for self-nurturing, exercise, and relaxation.

Too many possessions create stress and drain

your energy just by the need to take care of them. As you are able, pare your possessions down to the essentials, and to those things that bring beauty and meaning to your life. Make your home a refuge that is peaceful and beautiful. Everything in your surroundings affects you, so consciously create an environment that is deeply satisfying and relaxing.

## Cultivate the Art of Conscious Living

By cultivating your conscious moment-to-moment awareness, you have the opportunity to make adjustments throughout the day to keep your body relaxed and your mind calm. When you awaken in the morning, instead of immediately jumping out of bed, take a few minutes to begin your day in a peaceful way. Gently stretch your muscles, take a few deep, relaxing breaths, and visualize yourself moving through your day in a relaxed and conscious way. Throughout the day, pause every hour to stretch and take a few deep breaths to keep your energy flowing freely. Before bed, take time to relax in a warm bath, and sip a cup of chamomile or other calming herbal tea.

## Herbal Help for Stress and Anxiety

Herbs are valuable allies for relieving the symptoms of stress and also for enhancing resistance to stressors. Tonic herbs, such as American ginseng (*Panax quinquefolius*), Siberian ginseng (*Eleutherococcus senticosus*), and ashwagandha (*Withania somnifera*) help to strengthen the adrenal glands, which play a key role in helping the body adapt more easily to stressors. These herbs help to restore vitality, increase energy, and improve mental and physical performance. They also moderate the detrimental effects of stress on the body. You'll find more information on these beneficial herbal tonics in Chapter 8.

Sedative herbs are useful for relieving the symptoms of stress. Gentle herbs such as catnip (*Nepeta cataria*), chamomile (*Matricaria chamomila*), or lemon balm (*Melissa officinalis*) may be sufficient for mild tension and make pleasant-tasting beverage teas. To make a tea, pour one cup of boiling water over two to three teaspoons of dried herb. Cover, and steep for fifteen minutes. Strain, sweeten if desired, and drink up to three to four cups a day.

More powerful stress-relieving sedative herbs that are helpful during periods of intense anxiety include kava (*Piper methysticum*), passionflower (*Passiflora incarnata*), and valerian (*Valeriana officinalis*). They are discussed in detail in Chapter 9.

## CHAPTER 6

# NUTRITION FOR ENERGY AND HEALING

The old adage, "You are what you eat," is particularly appropriate in relation to how energetic you feel. In this chapter, you'll learn about the foods that support optimal energy production, and you'll also learn how to identify foods that may be taxing your body and contributing to fatigue.

## Eating for Energy

The foods you eat have an immediate and profound affect on your health, energy, and mood. When you eat a healthy, nutrient-dense diet, you're giving your body the fuel it requires to meet the tasks of daily life, as well as providing healing nutrients for maintenance and repair. If you suffer from fatigue, chronic fatigue syndrome, or fibromyalgia, it's particularly important to pay close attention to your diet.

A simple way of approaching dietary change is to center your diet on foods that are nutrient dense, and to minimize the foods that deplete your energy. In addition, recent research shows that chronic inflammation, caused in large part by dietary factors, plays a role in many degenerative illnesses, including chronic fatigue and fibromyalgia.

## Create a Nutrient-Dense Diet

Fresh, minimally processed foods are rich in a variety of essential nutrients, including the trace compounds that are necessary for optimal health. A healthy, balanced diet consists of fresh vegetables and fruits, lean proteins such as poultry, fish, and eggs, low-fat dairy products, legumes, whole grains, and the healthful fats found in extra-virgin olive oil, nuts, seeds, and avocados. Eating a wide variety of foods provides your body with the vitamins, minerals, antioxidants, essential fatty acids, and phytonutrients necessary for optimal health.

**Phytonutrients**
*Compounds found in plants that have protective, disease-preventing properties.*

Fresh vegetables and fruits offer a wide range of antioxidants and phytonutrients that help to prevent disease. Make it a goal to eat seven servings of vegetables daily. Fresh fruits satisfy the desire for sweets, but to keep blood sugar levels stable, eat no more than two to three servings daily, and choose low-sugar fruits such as grapefruit and berries over high-sugar fruits such as grapes.

Protein is essential for maintaining healthy organ function; it also helps to keep blood sugar levels stable. Eat approximately three to four ounces of protein at every meal, choosing from lean proteins such as fish, poultry, lean cuts of meat, eggs, dried cooked beans, legumes, and soy foods such as tempeh and tofu.

Healthful fats, such as those found in extra-virgin olive oil, nuts, seeds, avocados, and cold-water fish, help to balance blood sugar levels by slowing the release of glucose into the bloodstream. Healthy fats are also necessary for the production of prostaglandins, hormone-like substances that play a role in helping to control inflammation.

Avoid unhealthy fats, including polyunsaturated oils, hydrogenated oils, and excessive amounts of saturated fats. These fats trigger degenerative changes in cells, and are a primary cause of inflammation and degenerative disease. Polyunsaturated oils are found in safflower, corn, sunflower, and most other vegetable oils. Hydrogenated oils include margarine and shortening. Saturated fats are found in red meat and whole-milk dairy products.

In addition to eating a healthy diet, be sure to drink plenty of pure water each day. Dehydration is a common cause of fatigue. To stay well hydrated and maintain healthy organ function, we need about two quarts of fluids daily. About half of your need for fluids is provided in the foods that you eat, especially if you consume plenty of vegetables and fruits. Pure spring water or filtered water is the best option for supplying the rest of the fluids that your body needs. Get into the habit of drinking four to six glasses of water daily, preferably between meals.

Whenever possible, buy organically grown and processed foods and drink pure water. Conventionally produced foods are treated with a wide array of pesticides, hormones, antibiotics, and other chemicals. These compounds are stored in body tissues, causing toxic overload that contributes to fatigue and chronic degenerative illnesses.

## Why You Should Eliminate Sugar and Refined Carbohydrates

Keeping blood sugar levels stable is essential for increasing energy and vitality. One of the most important steps you can take to keep your blood sugar on an even keel is to stop eating sugar and refined carbohydrates.

When you eat sugar or refined carbohydrates, blood sugar (blood glucose) levels increase. This stimulates the pancreas to secrete insulin, triggering the uptake of glucose by the cells and thus returning blood sugar to normal levels.

If your cells are subjected to frequent assaults of sugar and simple carbohydrates, they can lose their ability to respond appropriately to insulin, a condition known as insulin resistance. When this happens, glucose levels remain at a high level in the blood while the pancreas continues to pump out insulin. When the cells finally get the message to start absorbing glucose, blood sugar plummets. Fluctuating blood sugar levels not only cause fatigue, but are linked to a wide variety of degenerative diseases, including chronic fatigue and fibromyalgia.

**Insulin Resistance**
*A condition caused by excessive sugar intake; the cells lose their ability to respond appropriately to insulin.*

To prevent insulin resistance, avoid sugars (which can be disguised as sucrose, glucose, fructose, maltose, lactose, corn syrup, honey, maple syrup, and concentrated fruit juice sweeteners) and refined carbohydrates such as white bread, white rice, and refined pasta. Whole grains and other complex carbohydrates are better choices, because they don't cause steep rises in blood sugar. In addition, eat protein and fat with each meal, which slows the digestion of carbohydrates and minimizes fluctuations in blood sugar.

## Eliminate Caffeine to Prevent Fatigue

If you're fatigued, it can be tempting to rely on caffeine for a boost of energy. But caffeine over-stimulates the adrenal glands and places the body in a state of chronic stress, resulting in fatigue after the initial stimulant effect wears off. Caffeine is also a prime contributor to sleep disorders, which exacerbate fibromyalgia symptoms, and of course, fatigue.

Because caffeine is a potent drug, giving it up

usually means that you're going to suffer from withdrawal symptoms—primarily headaches and increased fatigue. To prevent debilitating symptoms, reduce your intake of coffee and caffeinated substances gradually. For example, if you currently drink two cups of coffee each morning, cut back to one cup. Or substitute a mixture of half regular coffee and half decaffeinated, gradually increasing the proportion of decaf over a period of several weeks. Other sources of caffeine to eliminate include black tea, cola drinks, chocolate, coffee-flavored ice creams and candies, and some over-the-counter and prescription drugs, especially pain relievers, cold medicines, and menstrual cramp medications—check the labels for caffeine content.

## Inhibit Inflammation with Diet

A special consideration for people suffering from chronic fatigue and fibromyalgia is the role that inflammation plays in the disease process. Inflammation is a part of the body's normal healing response to injury or infection. But chronic inflammation has recently been recognized as a factor in a variety of illnesses, including chronic fatigue and fibromyalgia.

Chemical messengers called cytokines play an essential role in regulating the immune system and are responsible for the inflammatory response, which helps the body fight off infection. But if cytokines go awry, they can cause inflammation to go into overdrive, which creates a wide variety of degenerative conditions. For example, heightened cytokine activity is known to cause joint damage in rheumatoid arthritis, and researchers are just beginning to understand the other types of havoc that cytokines can cause. In addition to inflammation, cytokines can cause fever, fatigue, and achiness, all characteristic symptoms of chronic fatigue and fibromyalgia.

**Cytokines**
*Chemical messengers that help regulate immune function and play an important role in inflammation.*

In a study published in the July 2001 issue of the journal *Rheumatology*, researchers found altered cytokine production in patients with fibromyalgia, noting that the production of cytokines increased with the duration of the illness.

Dietary modifications are one of the most effective ways of suppressing inflammatory cytokines. Essential fatty acids, including omega-3 fats, and gamma linolenic acid (GLA) (found in evening primrose oil and borage oil) are some of the most helpful nutrients; vitamins B, C, E, and K are also beneficial for reducing inflammation. Omega-3 fats are found in cold-water fish such as salmon, trout, and sardines; flaxseeds, flaxseed oil, and walnuts are also good sources.

To help reduce inflammation, eat a serving of cold-water fish at least three times a week, and include a tablespoon of flaxseeds (or flaxseed oil) in your daily diet. Eating lots of fresh vegetables and fruits every day provides vitamin C, vitamin K, and the phytochemicals that help prevent inflammation. Essential supplements for curbing inflammation include the B-complex vitamins (25–50 mg daily), vitamin C (500 mg daily), vitamin E (400–800 IU daily), and GLA (240 mg daily) in the form of evening primrose or borage seed oil.

To prevent inflammation, avoid the overconsumption of omega-6 fatty acids (found in polyunsaturated fats), saturated fats (found primarily in red meat and full-fat dairy products) and strictly avoid hydrogenated fats and foods containing trans-fatty acids (found in shortening, margarine, and many processed chips, crackers, and baked goods). Because sugar and refined carbohydrates contribute to inflammation by triggering insulin surges, this is another compelling reason to avoid these foods.

## Supplements for Optimal Health

Even if you consistently eat a balanced diet, it's difficult to obtain optimal amounts of every nutrient. While supplements can't replace a healthy diet, they are essential for building energy and vitality and as part of an overall program for healing from chronic fatigue and fibromyalgia.

Take supplements with meals, because food enhances absorption and lessens the possibility of stomach upset.

### High-Potency Multivitamin/Mineral

Choose a high quality supplement that provides a wide range of all of the basic vitamins and minerals. If you are a man or a postmenopausal woman, do not take a supplement that contains iron, because it can accumulate to dangerous levels in the body and is implicated in cancer and heart disease.

### B-Complex Vitamins

B-complex vitamins are essential for energy production and for inhibiting inflammation. Buy a multivitamin that contains 25–50 mg per day of vitamins $B_1$, $B_2$, $B_3$, $B_5$, and $B_6$, plus 400 mcg of folic acid.

### Vitamin C

Vitamin C is necessary for energy production and also helps to prevent inflammation. Take 500 mg daily.

### Vitamin E

Vitamin E helps to improve glucose metabolism and decreases blood insulin levels. Choose the natural form (d-alpha) and take 400–800 IU daily.

## Chromium

Chromium improves the sensitivity of cells to insulin, which helps to keep blood sugar on an even keel and reduces cravings for sugar and refined carbohydrates. Take 200–600 mcg of chromium in the form of chromium picolinate daily.

## Calcium

Calcium calms the nervous system and has a sedative effect. Take 800 mg daily, or 1,200 mg if you do not eat many calcium-rich foods. Calcium citrate is the most easily absorbed form—for best assimilation, divide into two doses and take with meals.

## Magnesium

Magnesium is essential for carbohydrate metabolism and is also a muscle and nervous system relaxant. Take 400–600 mg daily in the form of citrate, malate, aspartate, gluconate, or lactate. Taking more than 600 mg daily can cause diarrhea.

## Gamma Linolenic Acid (GLA)

Gamma linolenic acid is essential for the production of prostaglandins, hormone-like compounds that decrease inflammation. Take 240 mg daily in the form of evening primrose or borage oil.

## Food Sensitivities and Fatigue

If you are experiencing recurring fatigue, chronic fatigue syndrome, or fibromyalgia, you may be suffering from undiagnosed food sensitivities. In some people, foods that are normally considered healthy foods—such as eggs, milk, or wheat—can cause fatigue, muscle and joint pain, digestive disturbances, headaches, insomnia, and other symptoms of CFIDS and fibromyalgia. If you are sensitive to certain foods, your body reacts to the food as though it were a toxin.

Although the idea of food intolerance or sensitivity is dismissed by many conventional medical doctors, many people report feeling significantly better when they avoid certain foods.

Testing for food sensitivities is often challenging; laboratory tests are generally expensive and may not provide accurate results. The best way to determine whether or not you are sensitive to specific foods is to follow an elimination diet. To establish a baseline, begin by keeping a food journal for three days, recording everything you eat as well as any symptoms you are experiencing. Then eliminate the most common allergens from your diet: milk and all dairy products, wheat, corn, citrus, peanuts, eggs, soy, and all processed foods containing artificial colorings and preservatives. In addition, it's helpful to eliminate caffeine, chocolate, and sugar because these substances are often underlying causes of fatigue.

If you are sensitive to any of these foods, you'll typically notice a reduction in your symptoms after one week of following the elimination diet. To determine which foods are triggering your symptoms, begin reintroducing the foods you have eliminated back into your diet one at a time. Choose one food, include it in your diet for three days in a row, and note any symptoms. If a food causes symptoms, don't continue eating it. Continue adding the foods you have eliminated back into your diet, giving each one a three-day trial, until you have tested each food.

Once you have determined the foods that cause symptoms, avoid the problematic food for at least three months. After that time, you can try reintroducing the food into your diet. Often, the food can be eaten without triggering symptoms, because food sensitivities frequently arise when certain foods are eaten repeatedly over a long period of time. Many people tend to eat the same foods day after day, with little variation. To prevent the development of future food sensitivities, make it a point to eat a wide variety of foods, and try to avoid eating the same food more than once every two or three days.

## CHAPTER 7

# ESSENTIAL SUPPLEMENTS FOR OVERCOMING FATIGUE

**I**n addition to the basic supplements discussed in Chapter 6, specific dietary supplements play a key role in helping you to recover from fatigue, chronic fatigue, and fibromyalgia. Some of these nutrients, such as alpha-lipoic acid, $CoQ_{10}$, and NADH, support the production of energy within cells. In many studies, researchers have found that the symptoms of chronic fatigue and fibromyalgia are the result of faulty cell metabolism. Other nutrients, including 5-HTP and melatonin, support the production of serotonin, the body's natural feel-good chemical; research shows that people suffering from chronic fatigue and fibromyalgia have decreased levels of serotonin.

**Serotonin**
*A chemical produced by the body that has calming and mood-enhancing effects.*

## Alpha-Lipoic Acid

A vitamin-like compound, alpha-lipoic acid is a potent antioxidant that also helps the cells to process energy. In the late 1980s, scientists discovered that this unique nutrient prevents cell damage by free radicals, and is actually more powerful than vitamins C and E when it comes to protecting cell health. Unlike other antioxidants, which are either water soluble and effective only inside of cells, or fat-soluble and work only within fatty cell membranes, alpha-lipoic acid is soluble in both water and fat. This means alpha-lipoic acid can effectively neutralize free radicals in every cell of the body. As an added benefit, alpha-lipoic acid enhances the effectiveness of other dietary antioxidants. This powerful nutrient also supports the B-vitamins in creating energy from carbohydrates, proteins, and fats; increases cellular levels of ATP (adenosine triphosphate—the chemical form of energy in cells); and helps to stabilize blood sugar levels.

**Free Radical**
*An unstable molecule produced by toxins or metabolic processes; a primary cause of degenerative disease and aging.*

Because of its role in cellular energy production, alpha-lipoic acid can be helpful for the treatment of chronic fatigue. The fact that it is an extremely powerful antioxidant also makes it useful for increasing overall health and well-being in chronic illnesses.

The body generates small amounts of alpha-lipoic acid, but most of the nutrient is obtained through diet (spinach and beef are good sources). However, to obtain the amounts necessary for treating specific ailments, supplements are necessary. Alpha-lipoic acid is available in capsules or tablets. It can be taken with food or between meals and is regarded as very safe at recommended doses. For treating chronic fatigue, the recommended dosage is 100–200 mg daily.

**Antioxidant**
*Protective substances that prevent cellular damage by free radicals.*

## L-Carnitine

An amino acid-like compound, L-carnitine is essential for the production of energy in the body. It carries fatty acids into the mitochondria—the part of the cells that converts fat into energy for the heart and muscles. Approximately 75 percent of L-carnitine is supplied by diet (red meat and dairy products are the richest sources), while the rest is made by the liver from a variety of nutrients. However, if the liver isn't functioning optimally or if dietary sources are lacking, it's easy to become deficient in this important nutrient.

Fatigue and muscle pain are typical symptoms of L-carnitine deficiency, which led researchers to theorize that supplementing with the amino acid could be an effective treatment for chronic fatigue syndrome and fibromyalgia. In a study reported in 1997 in the journal *Neuropsychobiology*, twenty-eight patients with chronic fatigue syndrome were treated with L-carnitine. Researchers found that twelve of the eighteen symptoms measured showed statistically significant improvement, and there was no worsening of any symptoms. The greatest improvement took place between four and eight weeks of treatment.

When buying carnitine as a supplement, buy only supplements labeled as L-carnitine, which is the form that is closest to that produced naturally by the body. For treating chronic fatigue or fibromyalgia, take 500–1,000 mg two times daily on an empty stomach. L-carnitine is safe, and there are no known drug interactions associated with the supplement.

## Coenzyme $Q_{10}$

Commonly known as $CoQ_{10}$, this vitaminlike nutrient is essential for health and energy. Also called ubiquinone (because it is ubiquitous in all cells), $CoQ_{10}$ is a member of a family of compounds called quinones, which work together with enzymes that are necessary for various metabolic processes in the body.

$CoQ_{10}$ is an essential component of the mitochondria (the energy factories of cells) and plays an important role in cellular energy production. Within the cells, sugars and fatty acids from foods are processed by enzymes to produce adenosine triphosphate (ATP), the fuel used by every cell in the body. $CoQ_{10}$ helps the mitochondria burn fuel. It's found in especially high concentrations in cells that have greater energy needs, such as the heart and muscles.

**Adenosine Triphosphate (ATP)**
*Made from sugars and fatty acids; the fuel used by every cell in the body.*

Although almost every cell in the body produces $CoQ_{10}$, many people are deficient because of poor diet (they lack sufficient amounts of the nutrients necessary for manufacturing $CoQ_{10}$) and the natural aging process. A variety of foods contain $CoQ_{10}$—organ meats, salmon, sardines, and peanuts are particularly rich sources. But it takes two pounds of beef or two and one-half pounds of peanuts to obtain only 30 mg of $CoQ_{10}$. Consequently, many people don't get enough of this important nutrient.

Without adequate $CoQ_{10}$, the body runs short on fuel and energy plummets. When levels of $CoQ_{10}$ are increased in the diet, stamina improves and the muscles have the energy they need to function properly. For this reason, supplementing the diet with $CoQ_{10}$ can be helpful for treating chronic fatigue and fibromyalgia.

$CoQ_{10}$ is available in a variety of forms, including tablets, softgels, capsules, and liquids. Because $CoQ_{10}$ is a fat-soluble compound, supplements that have an oil base—such as gel capsules—tend to be the most effective form. For optimal absorption, take $CoQ_{10}$ with a meal containing some fat.

For treating chronic fatigue and fibromyalgia, take 100 mg daily. In general, it takes two to three months to see improvement. There are no known side effects from taking $CoQ_{10}$, even at high doses.

## Magnesium and Malic Acid

While it has long been known that magnesium is necessary for health, it's only recently that this important mineral has received the attention it deserves. Essential for the production of energy, magnesium is also required for the proper functioning of the muscles and nervous system. Magnesium is found in a wide variety of foods, such as dark leafy greens, legumes, nuts, and whole grains, but most people don't get sufficient amounts through their daily diets.

Because of its role in promoting healthy muscle function, magnesium can be helpful for relieving the stiff and painful muscles that occur with fibromyalgia. To facilitate absorption, some health practitioners recommend combining magnesium with malic acid, which also appears to be beneficial for chronic fatigue and fibromyalgia. Malic acid is needed for the efficient production of ATP, the body's fuel.

In a study reported in the *Journal of Nutritional Medicine*, twenty-four people with fibromyalgia were given either a placebo or 1,200 mg of malic acid combined with 300 mg of magnesium daily. Four weeks into the trial, the researchers found no significant difference between the placebo and malic acid/magnesium groups. However, the researchers then gave all of the participants the malic acid/magnesium combination for six months, increasing the dosage incrementally. At a dosage of 1,600 mg of malic acid and 400 mg of magnesium, participants experienced a significant improvement in symptoms.

Malic acid (derived from apples) is widely available in supplement form; it's commonly used as a food additive and is very safe. Magnesium is available in a variety of forms. Supplements are inexpensive, but it's important to choose one that is easily absorbed. The best are magnesium citrate, aspartate, carbonate, gluconate, or sulfate. For optimal results, take 1,200—2,400 mg of malic acid combined with 300–800 mg of magnesium daily. It can take four weeks or longer to see a significant response to the combination of malic acid and magnesium.

High doses of magnesium can cause diarrhea in some people, but this is more likely with magnesium oxide than other types. If you have severe heart disease or kidney disease, do not use supplemental magnesium without first consulting your doctor.

## NADH

Nicotinamide adenine dinucleotide, or as it's more simply known, NADH, is a coenzyme made from vitamin $B_3$ (niacin). Present in all cells, NADH plays an essential role in energy production by combining with glucose to stimulate the production of ATP (adenosine triphosphate), which is the chemical form of energy in cells. The more NADH a cell has, the more energy it produces.

Because NADH increases energy within cells, it can be helpful for relieving chronic fatigue and the fatigue caused by fibromyalgia. NADH was previously only available intravenously because stomach acids destroyed the compound before it could reach the cells. However, enteric-coated tablets are now available, making NADH easily available as an oral supplement.

In a study supported by the Food and Drug Administration, researchers at Georgetown University in Washington, D. C., gave twenty-six patients with chronic fatigue syndrome 10 mg of NADH daily. Of those taking NADH, 31 percent reported feeling more energetic and mentally alert while taking the supplement, compared to a meager 8 percent of those taking a placebo. While two-thirds of those taking NADH were not helped by the supplement, it's worth trying if you suffer from chronic fatigue or fibromyalgia.

For best absorption, take NADH on an empty stomach with water, and remain upright and walk around for twenty minutes or more after taking the supplement. While it's generally regarded as safe, doses larger than 10 mg daily can cause restlessness, insomnia, or anxiety in some people. To reduce the possibility of side effects, begin by taking a small dose of 2.5 mg daily for a week or two, and gradually increase the dosage over a couple of weeks until you are taking 5 mg twice daily.

## 5-HTP (5-Hydroxytryptophan)

5-hydroxytryptophan (5-HTP) is a special form of the amino acid tryptophan. In the body, 5-HTP is created when tryptophan is broken down to make serotonin, an important neurotransmitter that controls mood, eating behavior, and sleep.

**Neuro-transmitter**

*A compound that facilitates communication between nerve cells.*

The body makes 5-HTP from foods rich in tryptophan, such as chicken, turkey, and dairy products. Supplements of 5-HTP are made from the seed of an African plant called griffonia (*Griffonia simplicifolia*). Unlike many supplements, molecules of 5-HTP are small enough to pass through the blood-brain barrier, which allows them immediate access to the brain. Once in the brain, the molecules are converted into serotonin.

5-HTP is an important supplement for people suffering from chronic fatigue and fibromyalgia because of its effects on serotonin levels. If you have an adequate supply of serotonin, you'll feel calm, relaxed, and sleep well. With too little serotonin, you're likely to feel depressed, anxious, and irritable, crave sweets and high-carbohy-drate foods, and suffer from insomnia. The lower your level of serotonin, the more severe physical and emotional symptoms tend to be. 5-HTP has also been shown to increase levels of pain toler-ance in people suffering from fibromyalgia, who tend to have low levels of serotonin.

In a double-blind study of fifty people with fibromyalgia, those who took 100 mg of 5-HTP three times a day for thirty days reported a sig-nificant decrease in pain and number of tender points, improvement in sleep, and a reduction in morning stiffness, fatigue, and anxiety.

For treating fibromyalgia, begin by taking 50 mg of 5-HTP three times daily with food. If you don't see results within two weeks, increase the dosage to 100 mg three times per day. For treat-ing insomnia, take 100–300 mg of 5-HTP thirty to forty-five minutes before bed. Begin with the lower dosage, and if you don't see results within a few days, then gradually increase the dosage in 50 mg increments as necessary.

5-HTP occasionally causes mild nausea during the first several weeks of taking the supplement. Starting with a low dosage lessens the likelihood of nausea occurring, as does taking 5-HTP with food. You might also consider taking enteric-coated capsules or tablets, which decrease the potential for stomach upset.

5-HTP may intensify the effects of drugs that increase serotonin levels, such as some prescrip-tion antidepressants. Too much serotonin can cause symptoms such as agitation, rapid heart rate, high blood pressure, and confusion. Do not take 5-HTP if you are taking prescription antide-pressants or other drugs that raise serotonin lev-els (including migraine drugs in the triptan family) without first consulting with your doctor. If you are taking carbidopa, prescribed for Parkinson's disease, 5-HTP may cause skin changes similar to scleroderma. If you are pregnant or nursing, consult your healthcare practitioner before taking 5-HTP.

## Melatonin

A natural hormone produced by the body, melatonin plays an essential role in regulating sleep/ wake cycles. In fact, melatonin can be thought of as the body's natural sleep aid. The pineal gland, a pea-sized gland located at the base of the brain, is in charge of regulating the production of this important hormone; the ebb and flow of melatonin determines the body's circadian rhythm, or biological clock.

**Circadian Rhythm**
*The body's internal biological clock; regulated by the hormone melatonin.*

In numerous studies, melatonin has been proven to be an effective aid for sleep disorders. By helping to restore healthy sleep patterns, melatonin can be beneficial in the process of healing from chronic fatigue syndrome and fibromyalgia, which are often characterized by disrupted sleep. Supplementing with melatonin can help to improve sleep quality and restore normal sleep/wake cycles, which increases energy levels and helps to relieve the pain of fibromyalgia.

The production of melatonin is closely tied to the rising and setting of the sun. During the day, melatonin levels are so low that it's difficult to detect the hormone in the body. As night begins to fall, decreasing light triggers the pineal gland to begin secreting melatonin. Body temperature drops and alertness wanes as your body prepares for rest. As you sleep, melatonin production continues, peaking at about 2 A.M. in healthy young people and at about 3 A.M. in elderly people.

After peaking, melatonin levels quickly decline, signaling the body to prepare for awakening at daylight.

The rate at which melatonin is secreted (referred to as the melatonin pulse) affects many physiological and mental functions. For example, memory, decision-making, and clarity of thinking are all profoundly affected by a decrease in melatonin. Fatigue, insomnia, headaches, irritability, and reduced immunity are also common side effects when the biological clock is thrown off kilter. Many things can influence melatonin production, including jet lag, emotional stress, aging, and chronic illnesses such as fibromyalgia and chronic fatigue.

Many people have found that taking supplemental melatonin helps to reestablish a healthy circadian rhythm, which facilitates better sleep patterns and sounder sleep. Melatonin also appears to enhance alertness the following day, as well as lessening mid-afternoon fatigue.

Melatonin should always be taken at night—preferably before midnight, because that's when the pineal gland naturally secretes the hormone. For optimal results, take melatonin approximately thirty minutes before you wish to go to sleep. Dosages vary from person to person because of differences in the absorption and metabolism of the hormone. Most people experience results with dosages between 1 and 10 mg of melatonin. Start by taking 3 mg before bed. If you sleep well but are drowsy in the morning, cut the dosage in half. If, on the other hand, your sleep doesn't improve, increase your dosage by 3 mg each night until you are sleeping well and waking refreshed.

Melatonin has also been shown to be helpful for people who wish to wean themselves from conventional sleeping medications. In a double-blind study reported in 1999 in *Archives of Internal Medicine,* thirty-four people regularly using benzodiazepine sedatives were able to stop the drugs by taking 2 mg nightly of melatonin. If you are currently taking prescription sedatives and are interested in switching to melatonin, consult your doctor for advice.

Melatonin is regarded as a safe dietary supplement. However, taking too much can cause sleepiness the next day, headache, depression, or intestinal discomfort. It's best to start with a low dose, and to take more only if necessary. Taking melatonin long-term may affect other hormones in the body. If you're planning to take melatonin more than for a few weeks, it's a good idea to do so under the supervision of your doctor, who can monitor the effects. If you are pregnant or nursing, consult your doctor before taking melatonin.

## CHAPTER 8

# RESTORE YOUR ENERGY WITH HERBAL TONICS

**H**erbs can be remarkably beneficial for alleviating fatigue, CFIDS, and fibromyalgia. In this chapter, you'll discover how a special class of herbs called tonics can help to rebuild your energy reserves, enhance your immunity, and improve your overall well-being. When combined with a health-building diet, appropriate exercise, and sufficient rest, tonic herbs play an essential role in helping you to feel your best.

## Ancient Wisdom for Modern Life

From the beginning of time, people have sought substances from the plant kingdom to restore health, prolong life, and enhance energy. In the ancient traditions of Ayurvedic and Chinese medicine, tonics are esteemed as the highest form of herbal healing. Ayurvedic practitioners prescribe tonics for the renewal of body and mind, with the goal of enhancing spiritual awareness and delight in living. Similarly, Chinese herbalists prescribe tonics to strengthen resilience, improve organ function and metabolism, and to further the development of what the Chinese call "radiant health."

The attainment of spiritual awareness and radiant health are not common considerations in conventional Western medicine. The difference is one of philosophy; while Western medicine focuses on the eradication of disease, Eastern medicine emphasizes strengthening and balancing the health and energy of the individual. Consequently, a Chinese herbalist regards a tonic as a "superior" medicine because of its varied and numerous health-promoting attributes, and relegates herbs with antibiotic, pain-relieving, or other specific medicinal properties to the lower class of "inferior" medicines because they merely relieve symptoms. In keeping with the philosophy of treating the disease rather than the person, Western medicine holds symptom-relieving drugs in high esteem. The search for "magic bullet" drugs leaves little time or inclination to explore the more gentle tonics. But no "magic bullets" have been found to heal the most common ailments of our time, including the debilitating fatigue that brings more people to doctors' offices than any other ailment. This is where tonic herbs excel. By improving the functioning of the body at a cellular level, tonic herbs strengthen resistance to both external invaders and internal breakdowns.

There are certain criteria an herb must meet to qualify as a tonic: the herb must restore balance and strengthen the functioning of an organ or system without throwing another organ or body system out of balance. Tonic herbs facilitate these changes by a wide range of actions rather than just by one specific action. Of equal importance to the herb's active properties is its safety— a tonic herb must be non-toxic and non-habit-forming, even when taken over a long period of time.

In traditional Chinese and Ayurvedic medicine, the health-promoting benefits of tonics were discovered by keen observation throughout centuries of use. Western medicine prefers a scientific approach, and researchers worldwide are studying these herbs to quantify reputed attributes and identify active ingredients. In study after study, tonic herbs are proving to have significant positive benefits.

According to traditional Chinese and Ayurvedic medicine, the improvement in energy that comes from the regular use of herbal tonics is the result of a deeper internal shift toward health. Herbal tonics provide a safe way to restore balance, rebuild health and vitality, and promote longevity—all in the midst of the ever-changing and often stressful conditions of modern life.

To help restore energy and vitality, choose one or more of the tonic herbs discussed in this chapter. For optimal benefit, the herbs should be taken for a minimum of three months, and can safely be taken indefinitely.

## Ashwagandha (*Withania somnifera*)

Also known as Winter Cherry, ashwagandha has been used for centuries in Ayurvedic medicine as a rejuvenative tonic herb. Translated from Sanskrit, ashwagandha means "that which has the smell of a horse."

## The Benefits of Ashwagandha

Ashwagandha is believed to imbue those who take it with the vitality of a horse; consequently, the herb is often used by men hoping to restore sexual vitality and energy. But ashwagandha is equally appropriate for women. As the most frequently prescribed tonic herb in Ayurvedic medicine, ashwagandha is recommended for anyone suffering from weakness or debility, including fatigue caused by nervous tension and overwork.

In Ayurvedic medicine, ashwagandha has a stellar reputation; it's believed to increase energy and endurance, promote longevity, support sexual vitality, calm the mind, enhance mental function, rejuvenate the tissues, strengthen immune function, encourage restful sleep, and help the body overcome imbalances caused by mental or physical stress, poor diet, lack of sleep, or environmental toxins. The herb has also been used as an anti-inflammatory to relieve arthritis and joint pain.

## Scientific Support for Ashwagandha

Researchers believe that compounds in ashwagandha called withanolides are responsible for the herb's remarkable properties. These compounds have been extensively investigated, and although most of the experiments have taken place in test tube or animal studies, the results indicate that the herb clearly has anti-inflammatory, immune-stimulating, and adaptogenic benefits. Researchers have discovered that withanolides are very similar to ginsenosides, the compounds responsible for the health benefits of ginseng. In fact, ashwagandha is often referred to as "Indian ginseng."

**Adaptogen**
*An herb that helps the body adapt more easily to life stressors.*

In studies, ashwagandha has been shown to stimulate immune cell activity and to inhibit inflammation. Research has also shown the herb has mild sedative and muscle-relaxing properties. These findings support the herb's traditional use as a tonic to bolster stress resistance and enhance general health and well-being. In the August 2000 issue of *Alternative Medicine Review*, the authors evaluated the available research on ashwagandha to determine the chemical properties, therapeutic benefits, and potential toxicity of the herb. They determined that ashwagandha has anti-inflammatory, antioxidant, antistress, immune-enhancing, and rejuvenative properties. In addition, ashwagandha has little or no toxicity. Because it's not clear exactly how ashwagandha works, the researchers recommended that the herb be studied more extensively, particularly in clinical trials.

## How to Use Ashwagandha

Ashwagandha is available in powdered form, capsules, and as a liquid extract. A traditional dosage is 1–2 grams of the dried powdered root, taken three times daily. As a liquid extract, take one-half to one teaspoon three times per day. A typical dosage of a standardized extract is 100–200 mg twice a day. As with all herbal tonics, it generally takes at least one month of consistent use to see benefits from taking ashwagandha. For best results, take the herb for at least three months; you can safely take it indefinitely.

Ashwagandha is non-toxic and has no reported negative side effects. The herb has been used for centuries in India, where even children suffering from emaciation are given ashwagandha to build their strength and vitality. However, if you are pregnant, it's always a good idea to check with your doctor before using any herbs or supplements.

## Panax Ginseng (*Panax ginseng*)

Used for more than 5,000 years as a rejuvenative tonic in Asia, ginseng is probably the best-known herb in the world. The botanical name, *Panax,* is derived from the Greek word panacea, meaning "cure all." While scientists don't claim that ginseng actually cures every disease, hundreds of research studies confirm that the herb increases endurance, relieves fatigue, bolsters immunity, helps regulate cholesterol and blood sugar, and enhances mental function. The results of these studies also support the traditional use of ginseng as a "chi" (or vitality) tonic. In China, ginseng is routinely recommended as a restorative for the elderly and anyone in a weakened condition.

Two species of ginseng are commonly used as tonics: *Panax ginseng*, which grows in China, and *Panax quinquefolius*, or American ginseng, which is native to the northeastern United States. Both have similar properties; in fact, Native Americans used ginseng in much the same way as the Chinese, and American ginseng is highly prized in China.

## The Benefits of Ginseng

In research studies, ginseng has been proven to enhance physical and mental performance and to help protect the body against stress. Scientists have identified dozens of compounds in ginseng, collectively called ginsenosides, which appear to be responsible for the beneficial effects of the herb.

While there are many theories as to how exactly ginseng works, many researchers believe that ginseng positively influences hormonal reactions, particularly those related to the body's stress response (commonly referred to as the "fight-or-flight" response). In daily life, we're all exposed to a variety of stress-inducing factors, from environmental stressors such as cold temperatures to emotional stressors such as fear, anxiety, and time pressures. Studies have shown that ginseng helps to lower levels of stress hormones called glucocorticoids, both immediately after stressful incidents and also during periods of prolonged stress. In addition, ginseng helps to strengthen the adrenal glands, improve the ability of cells to use oxygen, and moderate the wear-and-tear on the body caused by stress.

## Scientific Support for Ginseng

In a 1996 study reported in *Phytotherapy Research*, 232 subjects suffering from long-term fatigue participated in a double-blind forty-two-day clinical trial. All participants were given a multivitamin/multimineral supplement; half were also given 40 mg of a standardized extract of ginseng daily (the rest were given a placebo). The participants evaluated their symptoms on the first, twenty-first, and forty-second days of the study; at the end of the trial, only 5.7 percent of those taking ginseng reported fatigue symptoms, compared to 15.2 percent of those taking the placebo. Many animal and human trials demonstrate equally significant benefits from taking ginseng.

**Standardized Extract**

*An herbal product guaranteed to contain a specified amount of the herb's primary active ingredients.*

In another double-blind study reported in a 1994 issue of *Current Therapeutic Research*, researchers found that 205 people given a standardized ginseng extract (combined with vitamins and minerals) experienced significant improvement in various measures of quality of life compared to 185 people given a placebo. The researchers found the greatest benefits occurred in improvement in mood, vitality, and alertness; the patients with the lowest initial quality of life scores experienced the most improvement.

## How to Use Ginseng

Ginseng is widely available in a variety of forms, including as a liquid extract, powder, capsule, and tablets. Standardized extracts provide a guaranteed amount of ginsenosides, which have been identified as the active ingredients. Most clinical studies have used ginseng extracts standardized to 4% ginsenosides, at a dosage of 200–500 mg daily. If you are taking a nonstandardized preparation, it's best to follow the manufacturer's recommended dosages, because potencies vary greatly. A general dosage for non-

standardized preparations is 1–4 grams of pow-
dered root daily or $\frac{1}{4}$ to $\frac{1}{2}$ teaspoon daily of
liquid extract. Traditionally, ginseng is used cyc-
lically; for example, take the herb for two weeks,
and then take a two-week break before resuming
the dosage.

## Cautions for Ginseng

When used as directed at recommended dosages, ginseng rarely causes side effects. However, Chinese ginseng has been known to cause
irritability or hypertension in some people. If this
occurs, lower the dosage or switch to American
ginseng, which is less likely to cause over-stimu-
lation. Don't take larger than recommended doses
of ginseng, and do not use ginseng in combination with other stimulants such as caffeine.

## Siberian Ginseng
## (*Eleutherococcus senticosus*)

Also known as eleuthero, Siberian ginseng is not
actually a true ginseng, although it's in the same
botanical family as *Panax ginseng*. Indigenous to
Siberia and northeastern China, eleuthero has
been used for at least 2,000 years to improve
general health, increase energy, and prolong life.
Many studies have shown the herb to be an
invaluable aid for enhancing resistance to stress,
and people who regularly take Siberian ginseng
report an increased sense of psychological as
well as physical well-being.

## How Siberian Ginseng Works

The health promoting benefits of Siberian ginseng have largely been researched and docu-
mented by Russian scientists, who became
interested in the root of the spiny shrub as an
alternative to the more costly *Panax ginseng*. In
more than 1,000 studies, Siberian ginseng has

been shown to significantly increase energy and endurance for both physical and mental tasks, enhance immune function, and protect the body against environmental stressors and toxins. The herb also has been shown to normalize blood pressure, lower cholesterol, regulate blood sugar, and strengthen the adrenal glands.

Scientists have identified compounds in Siberian ginseng called eleutherosides, which have similar effects to the ginsenosides found in *Panax ginseng*. Many herbalists regard Siberian ginseng to be more appropriate for a wider range of people than the more stimulating *Panax ginseng*. The herb is approved by the German Commission E as a tonic for invigoration and fortification in times of fatigue or debility.

## How to Use Siberian Ginseng

To be certain of obtaining high-quality Siberian ginseng, look for products that are standardized for eleutherosides, which have been identified as the active ingredient. Products are typically standardized to contain at least 0.8% eleutherosides. Follow the manufacturer's recommendations, or take approximately 200–400 mg daily.

For best results, take Siberian ginseng for at least three months, with a two-week break before resuming the dosage. Considered to be safe and non-toxic, Siberian ginseng generally has no negative side effects and can be taken long-term with only positive benefits. While Siberian ginseng can help regulate blood pressure, if you have high blood pressure, consult your doctor before taking the herb. To avoid possible restlessness, avoid taking Siberian ginseng in the evening.

## CHAPTER 9

# HERBS FOR SYMPTOM RELIEF

**I**f you've been diagnosed with chronic fatigue syndrome or fibromyalgia, you've probably been given medications to help to relieve your symptoms. The most common medications for these conditions are pain relievers, sedatives to help you sleep, or drugs to ease anxiety and depression. Many of these prescription drugs may have unpleasant side effects, such as excessive drowsiness or digestive disturbances. Herbs offer an alternative for alleviating symptoms; they work in much the same way as drugs, but are less likely to cause unpleasant side effects. Many times, herbs can provide the extra support that can help bring the body and mind back into balance, without dangerous side effects, and without the risk of addiction.

## Kava (*Piper methysticum*)

Kava, a member of the pepper family, has been cultivated for centuries in Polynesia, where it is used as a ceremonial herb; it's also enjoyed as a social relaxant in much the same way that alcohol is used in the West. The root of the plant contains compounds called kavalactones, which have a mild tranquilizing effect similar to Valium. However, kava is not addictive, and in normal doses, it creates feelings of well-being instead of sedation. In contrast to prescription tranquilizers, kava calms the mind without affecting the ability to concentrate.

## The Medicinal Uses of Kava

In Western herbalism, kava is primarily used for treating anxiety, stress, and insomnia. Because the herb also acts as a gentle muscle relaxant and pain reliever, it can be helpful for chronic pain disorders such as fibromyalgia. Scientists are not certain as to exactly how kava exerts its sedative action but several theories have been proposed. Researchers have found that kava affects receptors in the brain called gamma-aminobutyric acid (GABA) receptors, which promote feelings of relaxation. Other studies have shown that kava acts on the limbic portion of the brain, which influences emotional responses. Kava has also been found to block the uptake of noradrenaline, a hormone that triggers the physiological stress response.

### Scientific Support for Kava

In numerous scientific studies, kava has been shown to effectively treat anxiety, stress, and insomnia. In a placebo-controlled study of 100 people diagnosed with anxiety, those who took 300 mg of kava extract daily for two months showed significant improvement in symptoms such as restlessness, heart palpitations, stomach upset, dizziness, and chest pain.

In a 1996 study of fifty-eight people suffering from general anxiety, participants were given either 100 mg of kava three times daily or a placebo. After one week, those taking kava reported alleviation of symptoms such as nervousness and tension; improvements continued throughout the four weeks of the study. Kava has also been found to be as effective as standard prescription anti-anxiety drugs. In a six-month, double-blind study of 174 people, kava was compared to two anti-anxiety drugs (oxazepam and bromazepam) and was found to relieve anxiety as successfully as the drugs.

## How to Use Kava

Kava is available in a wide variety of forms, including powdered extracts, liquid extracts, and capsules. The herb is often sold as a standardized extract, with the amount of kavalactones per dose listed on the label. For treating anxiety, the typical dosage is 40–70 mg of kavalactones three times per day. When taken specifically for insomnia, a dosage of approximately 180–210 mg of kavalactones thirty minutes before bedtime is appropriate.

For non-standardized kava products, the general recommended dosage is one 500 mg capsule up to three times a day, or fifteen to thirty drops of a liquid extract up to three times a day. For treating insomnia, the recommended dosage is two capsules or one-half teaspoon of liquid extract thirty minutes before bed.

Do not exceed recommended doses of kava and do not take kava for more than four weeks without consulting a qualified health practitioner. To prevent excessive sedation, kava should not be taken with prescription sedatives.

## Cautions for Kava

A growing number of reports in recent years have raised concerns about the safety of kava. In several cases, even at normal dosages, kava has apparently caused severe liver damage. Because of this, it's best to consult with a qualified herbalist or a healthcare practitioner familiar with herbs before using kava, especially if you plan to take it more than occasionally.

While kava has been implicated in at least a few cases of liver toxicity, there are many questions that remain unanswered. For example, the problem could be a result of the interaction between kava and other medications; those who have become ill could have had a preexisting liver disease such as hepatitis, or a high intake of alcohol could be a factor.

There's no question that kava is a valuable herbal medicine, and further studies are needed to determine what, if any, risk is actually associated with the herb. To be safe, follow these precautions, which are suggested by the American Botanical Council:

- Do not take kava if you have a history of liver problems without first consulting your physician.

- Do not take kava if you are taking any drugs (including over-the-counter drugs) that have known adverse effects on the liver.

- Do not take kava if you regularly consume alcohol.

- Do not take kava daily for more than four weeks without the advice of a qualified health-care practitioner.

- Stop using kava immediately and consult your physician if symptoms of liver toxicity occur, such as brown urine, yellowing of the eyes, nausea or vomiting, light-colored stools, unusual fatigue or weakness, stomach or abdominal pain, or loss of appetite.

## Passionflower (*Passiflora incarnata*)

A native tropical American plant, passionflower is an exotic vine with beautiful showy purple flowers. Used by the Incas as a tonic, the herb was brought to Europe in the late 1500s, where it quickly gained favor as a tasty beverage tea.

Today, passionflower is valued as a mild sedative, and is helpful for relaxing the muscles, easing nervous tension, and improving sleep quality.

## The Medicinal Uses of Passionflower

In America, early colonists found the Native Americans of the Gulf Coast using local passionflower as a tea for calming anxiety. By the mid-1800s, passionflower was regarded as an important remedy for insomnia and restlessness, and from 1916 until 1936, passionflower was listed as a sedative in the *National Formulary*, the reference guide for pharmacists.

Herbalists today use passionflower as a sedative and mild tranquilizer. In Europe, passionflower is a primary ingredient in natural tranquilizers and sedatives; the German Commission E, the equivalent of the United States Food and Drug Administration, lists passionflower as an approved treatment for "nervous unrest."

## Scientific Support for Passionflower

Research has shown that passionflower contains tranquilizing compounds, including passiflorine, which has similarities to the potent sedative morphine. In both animal and human studies, passionflower has been shown to have a sedative effect. In one study, French researchers gave ninety-one people suffering from anxiety either an herbal formula containing passionflower or a placebo. After twenty-eight days, those who were given the herbal formula reported a significant decrease in anxiety.

In a four-week, double-blind study of thirty-six people suffering from anxiety disorder, passionflower was found to be as effective as the prescription drug oxazepam in relieving anxiety symptoms. Oxazepam took effect more quickly, but by the end of the trial, passionflower was shown to be equally effective. The researchers also noted that passionflower did not cause side effects, such as impairment of job performance, that are typical of oxazepam.

### *How to Use Passionflower*

Passionflower makes a mild, good-tasting tea. Pour one cup of boiling water over one teaspoon of dried passionflower leaves. Cover, steep for ten to fifteen minutes, strain, and sweeten if desired. To relieve insomnia, drink one cup of tea thirty minutes before bed. For general anxiety, drink up to three cups throughout the day.

If you prefer, you can take passionflower as a concentrated liquid extract. Take $\frac{1}{4}$ to 1 teaspoon diluted in a small amount of warm water, up to three times a day.

### *Cautions for Passionflower*

Passionflower is considered safe in the amounts that are generally recommended. Pregnant women should not use medicinal amounts of passionflower, because compounds in the herb (harmala alkaloids) are uterine stimulants. If you are taking prescription sedatives, check with your health-care practitioner before taking passionflower because it may intensify the tranquilizing effects of the medication.

### St. John's Wort (*Hypericum perforatum*)

St. John's wort (*Hypericum perforatum*) was introduced to North America by early European colonists and now grows prolifically along roadsides throughout North America. A weedy-looking plant, St. John's wort is easy to overlook until mid-summer, when the plant bursts into bloom with tiny, yellow, star-shaped flowers. Throughout more than 2,000 years of use as a healing herb, St. John's wort has been valued for treating nerve injuries, inflammation, and burns. But the most compelling use that has brought St. John's wort to the forefront of herbal medicine has been the recognition of the herb's remarkable effects as a natural antidepressant.

### The Medicinal Uses of St. John's Wort

Since 1979, St. John's wort has been the subject of more than two dozen rigorous, double-blind, controlled clinical studies which have shown the herb to be as effective as pharmaceutical drugs for treating mild to moderate depression. St. John's wort has been found to relieve the sadness, irritability, anxiety, hopelessness, sleep disturbances, exhaustion, and other symptoms of depression as well as prescription antidepressants. As a result, St. John's wort is one of the most prescribed treatments for mild to moderate depression in Germany, and has become one of the top ten best-selling dietary supplements in the United States.

### How St. John's Wort Works

People suffering from depressive disorders typically have an imbalance of brain chemicals known as neurotransmitters; this imbalance triggers a variety of physical, emotional, and mental symptoms. Physically, these chemical imbalances manifest as changes in sleep, appetite, and energy. Emotionally, the person may feel a sense of hopelessness, irritability, or a lack of interest in work, socializing, or hobbies. And mentally, the person may have difficulties concentrating or making decisions. St. John's wort has proven helpful for alleviating all of these symptoms.

Researchers are still studying St. John's wort to determine exactly how it manages to alleviate depression. Some research indicates that the herb acts similarly to antidepressive drugs in that it inhibits the rate at which brain cells reabsorb serotonin (the neurotransmitter that acts as the body's natural feel-good chemical). People who are depressed often have low levels of serotonin. More studies are underway to determine precisely the active ingredients in St. John's wort, and to figure out exactly how these compounds work.

### Scientific Support for St. John's Wort

A number of studies support the use of St. John's wort for both depression and anxiety. An overview of twenty-three clinical trials published in the British Medical Journal found that St. John's wort extracts were significantly superior to a placebo in relieving depression, and just as effective as standard antidepressants. The studies involved a total of 1,757 outpatients with mild to moderately severe depressive disorders.

In a six-week German study, 240 patients suffering from mild to moderate depression were given either 500 mg of St. John's wort or Prozac every day. The patients were assessed using the Hamilton Depression Scale, a standard test used to measure depression. Both groups showed approximately a 12 percent decline in depressive symptoms at the end of the six-week trial. They were also tested using the Clinical Global Impression Scale, which showed that St. John's wort was significantly more effective in relieving depression than Prozac. Only six of the patients taking St. John's wort complained of side effects, and these were gastrointestinal symptoms. But thirty-four of the patients taking Prozac reported side effects, including gastrointestinal problems, vomiting, agitation, dizziness, and erectile dysfunction.

### Cautions for St. John's Wort

There are several advantages to using St. John's wort instead of pharmaceutical drugs: St. John's wort has far fewer side effects than drugs (and any side effects tend to be minor), St. John's wort extracts cost significantly less than pharmaceutical antidepressants, and patients tend to report greater satisfaction with St. John's wort than with drugs.

Most people can use St. John's wort safely, but as with any medicinal herb or drug, certain precautions should be observed. If you are taking prescription medications, consult with your doctor before taking St. John's wort because it may reduce the effectiveness of certain drugs. Do not take St. John's wort if you are pregnant without consulting your doctor.

If you are currently taking prescription medication for the treatment of a depressive disorder, do not begin taking St. John's wort without consulting your doctor. While many people have successfully switched from antidepressant drugs to St. John's wort, you should do so only under the supervision of your doctor.

### How to Buy St. John's Wort

St. John's wort is available in capsules, tablets, and liquid extracts.

All of the research on St. John's wort has been conducted using standardized extracts, which makes it easier for researchers to maintain consistency in their studies. Standardized extracts are herbal products that are guaranteed to contain a specified amount of what is believed to be the herb's primary active ingredient.

While St. John's wort products do not have to

be standardized to be effective, if you want to be certain that you are obtaining adequate levels of the active compounds, your best bet is to buy standardized extracts. St. John's wort extracts are typically standardized to contain 0.3% hypericin and 5% hyperforin.

### How to Use St. John's Wort

Most of the research on St. John's wort has used 900 mg daily of a standardized extract, taken as 300 mg three times a day. Some people notice a significant difference within a couple of weeks of taking St. John's wort, and report improvements in sleep quality, energy levels, and appetite. But for many people, it takes six weeks or longer to realize the full benefits of St. John's wort.

For most people, staying on the herb for at least one month after depressive symptoms have abated is helpful. Although there are generally no negative side effects associated with discontinuing St. John's wort, it's a good idea to taper off of it gradually, decreasing your dosage by 300 mg at a time over a period of weeks. While many people do take St. John's wort for brief periods, others find that they do best when they take the herb for months, or even years. St. John's wort can be taken for as long as is necessary and can be safely used for an indefinite period of time.

### Valerian (*Valeriana officinalis*)

Valerian has been used for more than 1,000 years for relieving muscle spasms, nervous tension, and insomnia. Brought to North America by early colonists, the plant now grows wild in much of the eastern United States and Canada. An attractive plant, valerian has fern-like foliage and clusters of tiny pale pink flowers in the spring. The strong-smelling root contains the compounds that give valerian its healing properties.

## The Medicinal Uses of Valerian

In the twelfth century, the noted German abbess and herbalist Hildegard of Bingen recommended valerian as a sleep aid. The plant was well regarded in this country up until the mid-1940s and the advent of pharmaceutical sedatives—in fact, valerian was listed in the *United States Pharmacopoeia* as a tranquilizer. While use in the United States declined, the popularity of valerian in Europe continued. Following numerous research studies, the herb was given official approval as a sleep aid by Germany's Commission E in 1985. France, Italy, Switzerland, and Belgium also approve valerian as an over-the-counter sedative.

Herbalists today routinely prescribe valerian for treating insomnia, anxiety, tension, and stress-related headaches and digestive disturbances. In treating chronic sleep disorders, valerian is most effective when taken consistently over an extended period of time. Studies have shown that valerian decreases the length of time that it takes to get to sleep, reduces the frequency of nighttime awakenings, eases nervous tension and anxiety, and improves overall sleep quality, all of which are helpful for people suffering from chronic fatigue and fibromyalgia.

## Scientific Support for Valerian

A number of studies, primarily by European researchers, have confirmed the use of valerian as a sleep aid. In five placebo-controlled studies and several large multicenter studies of more than 11,000 people, valerian has been proven to be an effective sedative and to improve sleep quality. In one German study, researchers gave 121 people suffering from insomnia valerian root extract or a placebo one hour before bedtime. A significant improvement in sleep quality was reported by the majority of participants who were given valerian. In another German study, sixty-eight adults suffering from chronic insomnia were given a combination of valerian and lemon balm extract or a placebo. Those who were given the herbal combination fell asleep more quickly, slept longer, and reported significantly greater feelings of well-being.

Other clinical studies have compared valerian to prescription sedative drugs. In a twenty-eight day double-blind trial of seventy-five people with insomnia, valerian was shown to be as effective as oxazepam, a benzodiazepine sedative. Additional studies have shown similar positive results.

Although valerian appears to be equally as effective as benzodiazepene sedatives, it doesn't share the dangerous side effects, such as impaired coordination, dizziness, and mood disturbances. Another benefit is that valerian is not addictive, nor does it cause the morning grogginess typical of prescription sedatives.

### How to Use Valerian

Valerian can be made into a tea, although many people find the strong, musky flavor unpleasant. If you want to make a tea, pour one cup of boiling water over one teaspoon of dried chopped root. Cover, and steep for ten minutes. Strain, and drink one cup thirty minutes before bed.

Valerian is readily available as a concentrated liquid extract or in capsules. Take one-half to one teaspoon of valerian extract thirty minutes before bed, or 300–500 mg of powdered root in capsules. It may take up to four weeks to stabilize sleep patterns. Studies have shown that the effectiveness of valerian increases over time.

### Cautions for Valerian

When used as directed, valerian is safe and rarely

causes side effects. As with any sedative, valerian should not be used if you are planning to drive or operate machinery within a couple of hours of taking the herb. Unlike prescription sedatives, valerian is not dangerous when combined with alcoholic beverages, but the herb can magnify the effects of alcohol. If you are taking prescription sedatives, check with your doctor before taking valerian. For a small percentage of people, valerian causes stimulation instead of sedation. If this occurs, switch to another sedative herb, such as passionflower.

## CHAPTER 10

# LIFESTYLE SUGGESTIONS FOR INCREASED ENERGY

**M**any times, it's the simple things you do that can be life changing. In this chapter, you'll learn about small changes you can make in your daily life that will help you sleep better, ease pain and stiffness, and feel more energetic.

## How to Get a Good Night's Sleep

Getting a good night's sleep is one of the most important things you can do to enhance your health and well-being. Spending time every night in the deep, restorative stages of sleep is essential for feeling refreshed and energetic, and studies have shown that the deepest stages of sleep are critical for relieving the pain of fibromyalgia. Because many lifestyle and environmental factors can interfere with a good night's sleep, addressing these issues is sometimes all that's needed to restore healthful sleeping patterns. If you need additional help, consider taking the supplement melatonin, which is discussed in detail in Chapter 7.

An erratic schedule is a common cause of sleep disorders. Working shift work or nights interferes with the body's natural sleep cycle, as does staying up too late on weekend nights and sleeping in on weekend mornings. In general, the body thrives on a regular schedule. Establish a specific time for going to bed and for getting up in the morning, and adhere to it as much as possible, even on weekends and during vacations.

It's also helpful to use your bed only for sleep and sex. Avoid watching television, working, studying, eating in bed, or making phone calls, because these activities stimulate alertness instead of allowing the body and mind to relax and prepare for sleep.

Regular, daily exercise is an excellent way of alleviating the stress that often interferes with sleep. In fact, studies have found that exercise is as beneficial as prescription drugs for promoting sleep. All forms of aerobic activity—including brisk walking, bicycling, and swimming—are effective for helping to overcome insomnia. As much as possible, exercise outdoors—particularly early in the day—to stimulate the production of hormones that promote restful sleep. In addition to moderate aerobic exercise, yoga and other gentle stretching and breathing exercises calm the body and mind and make it easier to go to sleep.

Many dietary factors play a role in helping to ensure a good night's sleep. It probably comes as no surprise that caffeine is at the top of the list of sleep disrupters. Make sure to avoid caffeine in all of its forms, including coffee, coffee-flavored ice cream and candy, black tea, colas, chocolate, and caffeine-containing drugs for weight loss, colds, and headaches. Alcohol can also cause sleep problems. A glass of wine with dinner can promote relaxation, but more than that can contribute to insomnia. An often-overlooked cause of restless sleep is hypoglycemia, which can give rise to middle-of-the-night awakening. To help keep blood sugar levels stable throughout the night, eat a snack that contains some protein, fat, and complex carbohydrates thirty minutes before bed, such as a few whole grain crackers with nut butter.

Creating a quiet, dark, and peaceful environment is necessary for a good night's sleep. If noise is a problem, wear comfortable earplugs or invest in a sound machine to mask bothersome noise. Light is also a primary environmental cause of sleep problems. Even a small amount of light resets the circadian rhythm and signals the body to wake up. Make your bedroom as dark as possible with blinds, shades, or drapes that block out all light. And make sure that your bedroom is a comfortable temperature—slightly cool temperatures promote the most restful sleep.

To help your body and mind prepare for a restful night's sleep, cultivate the habit of doing something relaxing in the hour before going to bed. Read a novel, listen to soothing music, meditate, or practice calming yoga poses. Soaking in a hot bath an hour or two before bedtime can also promote relaxation and help to ease muscle pain and stiffness.

If you find that you're still awake fifteen or twenty minutes after going to bed, don't lie there and fret about not sleeping. Instead, get up and go into another room to read, listen to soothing music, or engage in another quiet activity until you begin to feel sleepy. Don't watch television—it's too stimulating, and the bright light will trigger wakefulness. If for some reason you are physically unable to get out of bed, keep a boring book by the side of your bed and read by a low-intensity light.

## Exercise for More Energy

Although exercise may feel like the last thing you want to do when you're suffering from fatigue or pain, it's actually one of the best things you can do to restore your health and vitality. Exercise strengthens muscles, lubricates joints, and triggers the release of endorphins, the body's natural pain-relieving, feel-good chemicals. Regular physical activity also improves respiratory and circulatory function, stimulates lymphatic flow, enhances digestive function and elimination, strengthens the immune system, improves sleep quality, and helps relieve anxiety and depression.

In a British study, 55 percent of patients with chronic fatigue syndrome who participated in a twelve-week aerobic exercise program reported feeling much better with exercise. In a one-year follow-up, 74 percent of the participants maintained their improvement. Another study published in 1999 in the *Annals of Behavioral Medicine* showed that people suffering from fibromyalgia who exercised experienced significant improvement in both physical and psychological symptoms.

It's important to start slowly, and to exercise within your comfort zone. If you haven't been exercising, begin with a gentle ten-minute walk. Increase the walk by five minutes each week until you're walking thirty minutes or more at a time, five or more days a week. Make sure to exercise at a pace that is comfortable for you, and spend a few minutes stretching afterward to ward off muscle stiffness and soreness.

It's a good idea to vary your workouts to prevent overuse injuries. Aerobic activities strengthen the cardiovascular system and enhance circulation, improve lung capacity, oxygenate the cells, and increase the elimination of toxins. Stretching exercises, such as yoga, increase flexibility, calm the nervous system, and provide an internal massage, which improves the health of all of the organs and glands.

## Relaxation and Healing

Relaxation therapies such as breathing exercises, meditation, and visualization are useful for easing the muscle tension, pain, emotional stress, and insomnia that accompany chronic fatigue and fibromyalgia. When you're suffering from fatigue and pain, deep relaxation is an essential part of your healing process. By taking time every day to practice deep relaxation exercises, you calm and soothe your mind, release deeply held tension, and stimulate your body's healing energy.

Breathing exercises are a powerful method for relaxing your body, calming your mind, building vitality, and stimulating the flow of healing energy. By practicing even a few minutes of breath work, you immediately and positively influence your physical and emotional well-being. Set aside five or ten minutes every day to practice one or more of the following exercises. When you become familiar with conscious breathing techniques, you can practice them anywhere, at any time. You might find that you feel a bit light-headed when you first begin deep breathing practices. Be sure to work at a pace that is comfortable for you.

## Calming Breath

This simple exercise slows down your breathing, calms the mind, and helps to release tension.

- Sit in a comfortable position with your back straight, and focus your attention on your breathing.

- Inhale a slow, steady breath through your nose to a count of five, at a pace that is comfortable for you.

- Hold your breath for five counts.

- Open your mouth slightly, and exhale to a count of ten, keeping your exhalation smooth and controlled.

- Repeat the exercise for a total of five complete cycles.

## Vitality Breath

This breathing exercise helps to alleviate fatigue.

- Sit with your spine comfortably upright, your feet flat on the floor, and your shoulders relaxed.

- Inhale a series of rapid, short breaths through your nostrils until your lungs are completely filled with air.

- Exhale forcefully through your mouth, making the sound "ha" as you exhale completely.

- Repeat several times, and then resume normal breathing.

## The Benefits of Hydrotherapy

Hydrotherapy—or water therapy—is an excellent method for relaxing tense muscles and easing pain. A hot bath an hour before bed can promote restful sleep, and a hot morning shower can ease morning muscle stiffness and pain. Soaking in a hot Jacuzzi, mineral spring, or relaxing in a sauna are all also wonderful ways of easing tension, pain, and stiffness.

For a therapeutic bath, fill the tub with comfortably warm water. Add two cups of Epsom salts, which are rich in magnesium and help to relax the muscles and nervous system. For additional soothing benefits, add ten drops of lavender essential oil to the bathwater.

# CONCLUSION

As you've learned from reading this book, fatigue can be caused by a variety of factors, from diet and lifestyle to underlying physical conditions such as low thyroid function. Most of the time, simple fatigue can be remedied with lifestyle changes. Eating a healthier diet, exercising regularly, getting more sleep, and learning to relax provide your body with the basic necessities for building vitality. In addition, you can rebuild your energy and vitality more quickly by using the special nutrients and herbs discussed in this book.

The process of healing from fatigue—and especially chronic fatigue and fibromyalgia—can take a long time, and you'll probably experience some ups and downs in your journey. It's important to be patient and persistent, and to pay attention to what you discover best supports your well-being. Remember, too, that it can be very helpful to engage the help of a supportive and knowledgeable healthcare practitioner.

# SELECTED
# REFERENCES

Abraham GE, Flechas JD. Management of fibromyalgia: Rationale for the use of magnesium and malic acid. *Journal of Nutritional Medicine,* 1992; 3:49–59.

Archana R, Namasivayam A. Antistressor effect of Withania somnifera. *Journal of Ethnopharmacology,* 1999; 64:91–93.

Barbiroli B, Medori R, Tritschler H-J, et al. Lipoic (thioctic acid) increases brain energy availability and skeletal muscle performance as shown by in viv 31P-MRS in a patient with mitochondrial cytopathy. *Journal of Neurology,* 1995; 242:472–477.

Eisinger J, Plantamura A, Ayavou T. Glycolysis abnormalities in fibromyalgia. *Journal of the American College of Nutrition,* 1994 Apr; 13(2): 144–148.

Forsyth LM, Preuss HG, MacDowell AL, et al. Therapeutic effects of oral NADH on the symptoms of patients with chronic fatigue syndrome. *Annals of Allergy, Asthma, and Immunology,* 1999; 82:185–191.

Griep EN, Boersma JW, de Kloet ER. Altered reactivity of the hypothalamic-pituitary-adrenal axis in the primary fibromyalgia syndrome. *Journal of Rheumatology,* 1993 Mar; 20(3):469–474.

Jason LA, Richman JA, Rademaker AW, et al. A Community-Based Study of Chronic Fatigue Syndrome. *Archives of Internal Medicine,* 1999; 159(18):2129–2137.

LeGal M, Cathebras P, Struby K. Pharmaton capsules in the treatment of functional fatigue: a double-blind study versus placebo evaluated by a new methodology. *Phytotherapy Research,* 1996; 10:49–53.

Logan AC, Wong C. Chronic Fatigue Syndrome: Oxidative Stress and Dietary Modifications. *Alternative Medicine Review,* 2001; 6(5):450–459.

Lue FA. Sleep and Fibromyalgia. *Journal of Musculoskeletal Pain,* 1994; 2: 89–100.

Panda S, Kar A. Withania somnifera and Bauhinia purpurea in the regulation of circulating thyroid hormone concentrations in female mice. *Journal of Ethnopharmacology,* 1999; 67(2):233–239.

Patarca-Montero R, Antoni M, Fletcher MA, et al. Cytokine and Other Immunologic Markers in Chronic Fatigue Syndrome and Their Relation to Neuropsychological Factors. *Applied Neuropsychology,* 2001; 8(1):51–64.

Plioplys AV, Plioplys S. Amantadine and L-carnitine treatment of chronic fatigue syndrome. *Neuropsychobiology,* 1997; 35:16–23.

Tripathi YB, Malhotra OP, Tripathi SN. Thyroid stimulating action of Z-guggulsterone obtained from Commiphora mukul. *Planta Medica,* 1984; (1):78–80.

Wiklund I, Karlberg J, Lund B. A double-blind comparison of the effect on quality of life of a combination of vital substances including standardized ginseng G115 and placebo. *Current Therapeutic Research,* 1994; 55(1): 32–42.

# OTHER BOOKS AND RESOURCES

**The CFIDS Association of America**
www.cfids.org

**The National Fibromyalgia Association**
www.fmaware.org

**Centers for Disease Control and Prevention**
www.cdc.gov

Challem, J. *The Inflammation Syndrome: The Complete Nutritional Program to Prevent and Reverse Heart Disease, Arthritis, Diabetes, Allergies and Asthma*, NJ: John Wiley & Sons, 2003.

Challem J, Berkson B, Smith M. *Syndrome X: The Complete Nutritional Program to Prevent and Reverse Insulin Resistance*, NJ: John Wiley & Sons, 2000.

Vukovic, L. *Herbal Healing Secrets for Women*. Paramus, NJ: Prentice Hall, 1998.

Vukovic, L. *14-Day Herbal Cleansing*. Paramus, NJ: Prentice Hall, 1998.

Vukovic, L. *User's Guide to St. John's Wort*. NJ: Basic Health Publications, 2002.

**GreatLife Magazine**
Consumer magazine with articles on vitamins, minerals, herbs, and foods.
*Available for free at many health and natural food stores.*

### Let's Live Magazine

Consumer magazine with emphasis on the health benefits of vitamins, minerals, and herbs.

Customer service:

1-800-676-4333

P.O. Box 74908

Los Angeles, CA 90004

*Subscriptions: 12 issues per year, $19.95 in the U.S.; $31.95 outside the U.S.*

### Physical Magazine

Magazine oriented to body builders and other serious athletes.

Customer service:

1-800-676-4333

P.O. Box 74908

Los Angeles, CA 90004

*Subscriptions: 12 issues per year, $19.95 in the U.S.; $31.95 outside the U.S.*

### The Nutrition Reporter™ newsletter

Monthly newsletter that summarizes recent medical research on vitamins, minerals, and herbs.

Customer service:

P.O. Box 30246

Tucson, AZ 85751-0246

e-mail: jack@thenutritionreporter.com

www.nutritionreporter.com

*Subscriptions: 12 issues per year, $26 in the U.S.; $32 U.S. or $48 CNC for Canada; $38 for other countries.*

# INDEX

Printed in the USA
CPSIA information can be obtained
at www.ICGtesting.com
JSHW051956150824
68134JS00050B/51

9 781681 628479